CW00631388

MCQ Selftest Companion to Lee's Synopsis of Anaesthesia

G. B. Rushman

N. J. H. Davies

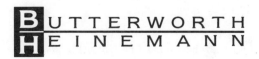

BUTTERWORTH
HEINEMANN

£ 12,99

Butterworth-Heinemann Ltd
Linacre House, Jordan Hill, Oxford OX2 8DP

◌ A member of the Reed Elsevier plc group

OXFORD LONDON BOSTON
MUNICH NEW DELHI SINGAPORE SYDNEY
TOKYO TORONTO WELLINGTON

First published 1995

© Butterworth-Heinemann Ltd 1995

All rights reserved. No part of this publication may be reproduced in
any material form (including photocopying or storing in any medium by
electronic means and whether or not transiently or incidentally to some
other use of this publication) without the written permission of the
copyright holder except in accordance with the provisions of the Copyright,
Designs and Patents Act 1988 or under the terms of a licence issued by the
Copyright Licensing Agency Ltd, 90 Tottenham Court Road, London,
England W1P 9HE. Applications for the copyright holder's written
permission to reproduce any part of this publication should be addressed
to the publishers

British Library Cataloguing in Publication Data
Rushman, G. B.
  MCQ Selftest Companion to Lee's
  Synopsis of Anaesthesia
  I. Title II. Davies, N. J. H.
  617.96076

ISBN 0 7506 2325 X

Library of Congress Cataloguing in Publication Data
A catalogue record for this title is
available from the Library of Congress

Typeset by Bath Typesetting Ltd, Bath
Printed and bound in Great Britain by Biddles Ltd, Guildford and King's Lynn

Contents

Preface

This companion volume to *Lee's Synopsis of Anaesthesia* has been developed to enable the reader to check how much of the factual information from the Synopsis has been retained. This does not, of course, cover the whole area of anaesthesia contained in the Synopsis, which includes much about the art of the subject, and the wisdom of many years of experience, both of which are difficult to test.

Nevertheless, the art of anaesthesia rests firmly on a database of scientific knowledge. Such background knowledge is most easily tested by the MCQ format, presented here. The questions have been carefully formatted in a friendly way, to help develop the reader's knowledge of the subject, and some of the questions are therefore slightly different from 'exam' questions. They are designed to augment what you have gleaned from your studies, rather than to test in a destructive or competitive sense.

This little book is unashamedly dedicated to improving the quality of anaesthesia. It is also dedicated to helping students of anaesthesia pass exams, which has been a long-term aim of the Synopsis itself!

On each question, there is the briefest reference to the page of the Synopsis to which the question refers. After each question, a brief explanation of the reason for a statement being false is frequently included. The answers on the right-hand side of the page may be covered up by a card or ruler, while the statement is assessed, and then checked against the reader's views.

The 'true or false' format has its limitations, since nothing is always true in medicine, nor is something always false, nor does something always happen, nor does something never happen. Our medical 'rules' are occasionally tested by exceptions, especially in the areas of intensive care and internal medicine, and we remember such exceptions. This is a minor drawback to the excellent value of the MCQ format, which enables the eagle-eyed critic to spot answers with which he may disagree. We have attempted to eliminate ambiguous answers in this book and encourage the reader to use it in this spirit.

GBR
NJHD

1 Physiology

Page 3

I The cell membrane:
1 Is freely permeable to urea
2 Is freely permeable to CO_2
3 Is a site for immune reactions
4 Is the site for the main action of thiopentone
5 Is the site for the action of muscle relaxants

Page 5

2 The acetylcholine-sensitive channels at the neuromuscular junction:
1 Are small proteins
2 Are blocked open by mivacurium
3 Are destroyed 2 weeks after major burns
4 Are blocked by calcium administration
5 Are absent in suxamethonium apnoea

Page 6

3 Acetylcholine:
1 Is antagonised by atropine in the CNS
2 Is highly lipophilic

3 Is enhanced by neostigmine in the CNS
4 Is blocked by pipecuronium at the muscarinic sites
5 Is a catecholamine

Page 7

4 Opioid receptors:
1 Mu receptors mediate analgesia at spinal cord level
2 Delta receptors are blocked by endorphins
3 Delta receptors are blocked by enkephalins
4 Have a high affinity for naloxone
5 Nausea and vomiting are mediated by mu receptors

Page 8

5 Sleep:
1 Tumescence of the penis occurs in NREM sleep
2 Respiratory rate is depressed in NREM sleep
3 Obstructive sleep apnoea occurs in REM sleep
4 NREM sleep is characterised by dreams
5 REM sleep is characterised by rapid low-voltage EEG

6 The Pickwickian syndrome is characterised by:
1 Obesity
2 Snoring

The cell membrane:
1 True
2 True (CO_2 is one of the most diffusible substances in the body)
3 True (many antigens are on cell walls)
4 True (probably at the GABA controlled chloride channel)
5 True (at the neuromuscular junction)

The acetylcholine-sensitive channels at the neuromuscular junction:
1 False (240,000 daltons)
2 False (they are blocked closed)
3 False (they proliferate as extrajunctional receptors)
4 False (calcium reverses neuromuscular blockade)
5 False (suxamethonium apnoea is a pharmacokinetic problem)

Acetylcholine:
1 True (this causes the anticholinergic syndrome)
2 False (its highly-ionised, highly-charged structure makes it lipophobic)
3 False (neostigmine does not cross the blood brain barrier)
4 False (it is blocked at the nicotinic sites)
5 False (it is a parasympathetic and neuromuscular transmitter)

Opioid receptors:
1 False (kappa receptors)
2 False (they are stimulated)
3 False (they are stimulated)
4 True (they have high affinity, but no efficacy)
5 True

Sleep:
1 False (in REM sleep)
2 True
3 True
4 False (dreams occur in REM sleep)
5 True

The Pickwickian syndrome is characterised by:
1 True
2 True

3 Restless sleep at night
4 Daytime sleep
5 Cafe au lait skin discoloration

Page 8
7 Potency of volatile anaesthetics:
1 Is directly related to lipid solubility
2 Is directly related to degree of fluorination of the molecule
3 Is directly related to blood solubility
4 Is inversely related to age in adults
5 Is inversely related to age in neonates

Page 9
8 Autoregulation of cerebral bloodflow:
1 Occurs below a mean arterial pressure of 100 mmHg
2 Occurs below a mean arterial pressure of 70 mmHg
3 Occurs below a mean arterial pressure of 50 mmHg
4 Is prevented by a reduction of $PaCO_2$ to 4 kPa
5 Is prevented by atropine

9 The pressure of the cerebro-spinal fluid:
1 Is 100–150 mmHg
2 Varies with arterial pulse
3 Varies with venous pressure
4 Influences intraocular pressure
5 Varies with $PaCO_2$

10 Cerebro-spinal fluid (CSF):
1 Has 5000 leucocytes per cu.mm
2 Is a transudate
3 Has a protein content of 40 g/l
4 Protein content rises in spinal analgesia
5 Spinal CSF volume in adults is about 70 ml

Page 10
11 The blood-brain barrier is normally easily crossed by:
1 Bupivacaine
2 Propofol
3 Desflurane
4 Penicillin
5 Mivacurium

3 True
4 True
5 False (skin is normal colour)

Potency of volatile anaesthetics:
1 True (Meyer–Overton theory)
2 False (e.g. desflurane has MAC 6%; halothane 0.8%)
3 False
4 False (the older the patient, the greater the potency)
5 True (the newborn is more sensitive to volatile agents than the 1 month-old)

Autoregulation of cerebral bloodflow:
1 True
2 True
3 False (this is the lower limit of normal autoregulation)
4 False (this $PaCO_2$ preserves autoregulation)
5 False (no effect)

The pressure of the cerebro-spinal fluid:
1 True
2 True
3 True (demonstrated in Queckenstedt's test)
4 True
5 True (a direct relationship)

Cerebro-spinal fluid (CSF):
1 False (< 5 per cu.mm)
2 False (an active secretion)
3 False (it has a protein content of 200–400 mg/l)
4 True
5 True

The blood-brain barrier is normally easily crossed by:
1 True
2 True
3 True
4 False (only crosses in meningitis)
5 False (muscle relaxants only cross in small amounts)

Page 10

12 **'A' nerve fibres:**
1 Transmit impulses at 10–120 m/sec
2 Are non-medullated
3 Are found in the white rami

4 The smaller ones recover first from local analgesics
5 Contain nodes of Ranvier

Page 12

13 **The substantia gelatinosa:**
1 Controls muscle co-ordination
2 Is influenced by TENS
3 Modulates pain transmission
4 Contains kappa receptors
5 Is a site of action of substance P

Page 14

14 **Sympathetic nerve fibres to the head:**
1 Arise from the upper 3 thoracic spinal cord segments
2 Synapse in the stellate ganglion
3 Travel with cranial nerves VIII–XII
4 Travel with carotid and vertebral arteries
5 Constrict the pupil

15 **Cardiac arrhythmias during anaesthesia are more frequent with:**
1 Sevoflurane
2 Rocuronium
3 Hyperkalaemia
4 Halothane
5 Hypotension

Page 16

16 **In the normal ECG:**
1 PR interval = 0.12–0.2 sec
2 QRS interval = < 0.1 sec
3 Q wave = < 0.04 sec except in leads III and aVR
4 The T wave is upright in V 3–6
5 The tallest R wave is less than 30 mm

17 **The PR interval in the ECG:**
1 Is from the end of the P wave to the start of the QRS
2 Indicates conduction time in the AV node and bundles of His

'A' nerve fibres:
1 True
2 False (these somatic fibres are all medullated)
3 False (white rami are the thoracolumbar autonomic outflow
        and have thinner 'B' fibres)
4 False (the small ones are blocked first and recover last)
5 True

The substantia gelatinosa:
1 False (it controls pain)
2 True (by closure of the 'gate mechanism')
3 True
4 True
5 True

Sympathetic nerve fibres to the head:
1 True
2 True
3 True
4 True
5 False (they dilate the pupil)

Cardiac arrhythmias during anaesthesia are more frequent with:
1 False
2 False
3 True
4 True
5 True

In the normal ECG:
1 True
2 True
3 True
4 True (indicates ventricular repolarisation)
5 True

The PR interval in the ECG:
1 False (start of P wave to the start of QRS)
2 True

3 Is normally not greater than 0.12 sec
4 Lengthens progressively in Mobitz type 2 heart block
5 May be prolonged by propofol

Page 17
18 The right ventricular preload depends on:
1 Blood volume
2 Venous tone
3 Respiration
4 Muscle activity
5 Posture

19 Myocardial contractility is influenced by:
1 Heart rate
2 Hypercapnia
3 Thiopentone
4 Dobutamine
5 Vitamin C

Page 18
20 The heart rate:
1 Increases in response to atrial stretch
2 Increases in inspiration
3 Is the main determinant of cardiac output in infants
4 Increases if intracranial pressure is raised
5 Increases if intraocular pressure is raised

21 Systemic vascular resistance:
1 Is normally about 1200 dynes.sec.cm^{-5}
2 Is directly related to cardiac output
3 Is decreased by haemodilution
4 Equals mean arterial pressure less central venous pressure divided by cardiac output
5 Is reduced in septic shock

Page 19
22 Coronary blood flow:
1 Is about 250 ml/min in the adult
2 Is greatest in systole
3 Is increased by beta agonists
4 Drainage is all through the coronary sinus
5 Supplies lactate to the myocardium

3 False (between 0.12 and 0.2 sec)
4 False (it does this in Mobitz type 1)
5 True (see Synopsis, page 171)

The right ventricular preload depends on:
1 True
2 True
3 True (greater venous pressure in expiration)
4 True (muscle pump causes venous return)
5 True (foot-up position aids venous return)

Myocardial contractility is influenced by:
1 True (the Bowditch effect)
2 True (increased in hypercapnia)
3 True (thiopentone reduces it)
4 True (a positive inotrope)
5 False

The heart rate:
1 True (the Bainbridge reflex)
2 True (sinus arrhythmia)
3 True (their cardiac output is very rate-dependent)
4 False (decreases)
5 False (eyeball pressure can be used to slow the heart)

Systemic vascular resistance:
1 True
2 False (inversely related)
3 True (by reducing blood viscosity)

4 True
5 True (see Synopsis, Chapter 33)

Coronary blood flow:
1 True
2 False (occurs in LV muscle only during diastole)
3 True
4 False (also via Thebesian veins)
5 True (a myocardial metabolic substrate)

Page 19
23 Systemic capillaries:
1   Are about 1 μm in diameter
2   Allow free protein transfer
3   Are dilated by CO_2
4   Are the primary site of pathology in septic shock
5   Have endothelium about 1 μm thick

24 The coronary arteries:
1   Are three in number
2   Are dilated by isoflurane
3   Are dilated by adenosine
4   Are dilated by prostacyclin
5   Are dilated by vagal stimulation

Page 21
25 The larynx:
1   Lies level with cervical vertebrae 3–6
2   The vestibule lies between the false cords and the aryepiglottic folds
3   The saccule is between false cords and vocal cords
4   The vocal cords are covered by ciliated epithelium
5   The glottis is closed by the extrinsic muscles

Page 22
26 The superior laryngeal nerve:
1   Is a branch of the tenth cranial nerve
2   Gives off the recurrent laryngeal nerve
3   Gives sensory supply below the vocal cords
4   Supplies the cricothyroid muscle
5   Gives sensory supply to the epiglottis

27 Granuloma after short-term intubation most commonly occurs:
1   At the carina
2   In the trachea
3   On the arytenoids
4   Anterior two-thirds of the cords
5   Posterior third of the cords

Page 23
28 The adult trachea:
1   Extends from vertebral levels C6 to T5
2   Has sensory supply from the vagus nerve
3   Has squamous epithelium

Systemic capillaries:
1   False (5–9 μm; red cell size 5–8 μm)
2   False (endothelial pores only 20–100 nm)
3   True
4   True (see Synopsis, Chapter 33)
5   True

The coronary arteries:
1   False (2 – right and left)
2   True
3   True
4   True
5   False (no effect)   *Gaseous : vagal shunt → dilatation*

The larynx:
1   True (in the adult, higher in children)

2   True
3   True
4   False (the trachea has ciliated epithelium)
5   False (intrinsic muscles)

The superior laryngeal nerve:
1   True
2   False (internal and external branches)
3   False (recurrent laryngeal does this)
4   True (via external branch)
5   True (via internal branch)

Granuloma after short-term intubation most commonly occurs:
1   False
2   False
3   False
4   False
5   True

The adult trachea:
1   True
2   True
3   False (ciliated)

4 Is supplied by the inferior thyroid artery
5 Is crossed by the aorta

Page 23
29 **The trachea:**
1 Nerve supply is from the recurrent laryngeal nerve
2 Is 1 inch (2.5 cm) long in the neonate
3 Is the narrowest part of the upper airway in the infant
4 Is a posterior relation of the innominate artery
5 Is surrounded by cartilages

Page 24
30 **The lungs:**
1 Biodegrade fentanyl
2 Are a site of action of angiotensin converting enzyme
3 Produce interleukin-1
4 Are rich in macrophages
5 Are a source of catecholamines

Page 25
31 **Oxygen consumption:**
1 Is reduced in early septic shock
2 Is increased in pyrexia
3 Is normally 3.5 ml/kg in the adult
4 Is reduced by volatile anaesthetics
5 Normally controls minute volume

Page 26
32 **Alveolar PO_2 is reduced by:**
1 Falling cardiac output
2 More than half at 18,000 feet of altitude
3 Hypercapnia
4 Nitrous oxide on induction of anaesthesia
5 Massive pulmonary embolism

Page 27
33 **Pulmonary shunt is increased by:**
1 Chest infection
2 Anaesthesia
3 Obesity
4 Smoking
5 ARDS

4 True
5 True

The trachea:
1 True
2 True
3 False (the cricoid cartilage)
4 True
5 False (cartilage rings are incomplete)

The lungs:
1 True
2 True
3 True
4 True
5 False (they biodegrade catecholamines)

Oxygen consumption:
1 False
2 True
3 True
4 True
5 False (blood CO_2 level does)

Alveolar PO_2 is reduced by:
1 False (falling cardiac output absorbs less O_2 from alveoli)
2 True
3 True (calculated by alveolar air equation)
4 False (increased – the reverse of the Fink effect)
5 False (less O_2 absorbed in pulmonary embolism)

Pulmonary shunt is inreased by:
1 True (by blocking small airways)
2 True (by closing alveoli)
3 True (by raising closing volume)
4 True
5 True

Page 28

34 The oxygen dissociation curve of haemoglobin is moved to the:
1 Right by hypercapnia
2 Left by decrease of 2,3-DPG
3 Left in carbon monoxide poisoning
4 Left by abnormal haemoglobins
5 Right during pregnancy

Page 30

35 Pulmonary vascular resistance is affected by:
1 Posture
2 Isoprenaline
3 Hypoxia
4 Prostacyclins
5 Acidosis

Page 41

36 Body water:
1 Is relatively higher in infants than in adults

2 Intracellular fluid osmolality is controlled by ADH
3 Osmolality of ECF is 275–300 mosmol/l
4 Osmolality of ECF is controlled by water balance
5 Volume of ECF is controlled by sodium balance

37 Aldosterone:
1 Is secreted in the adrenal medulla
2 Moves water to the intracellular compartment
3 Causes secretion of salt
4 Acts on the collecting ducts of the kidney
5 Is secreted in response to surgery

38 Antidiuretic hormone:
1 Is a peptide
2 Is inhibited by surgery and trauma
3 Alters urine osmolality between 30 and 1400 mosmol/l
4 Is secreted in response to a fall in extracellular osmolality
5 Is secreted in response to hypovolaemia

Page 42

39 Renal blood flow is controlled by:
1 Angiotensin
2 Sympathetic tone
3 Aldosterone

The oxygen dissociation curve of haemoglobin is moved to the:
1 True
2 True
3 True
4 True
5 True

Pulmonary vascular resistance is affected by:
1 True
2 True
3 True (a pulmonary vasoconstrictor)
4 True (pulmonary vasodilators)
5 True (a pulmonary vasoconstrictor)

Body water:
1 True (gives a higher volume of distribution
         for many drugs in infants)
2 False (extracellular fluid)
3 True
4 True
5 True

Aldosterone:
1 False (secreted in the zona glomerulosa of the adrenal cortex)
2 False
3 False (retention of salt)
4 True (and distal tubules)
5 True

Antidiuretic hormone:
1 True
2 False (secreted in response to surgery)
3 True
4 False (to a rise in osmolality)
5 True (a defence mechanism)

Renal blood flow is controlled by:
1 True
2 True
3 False

4 Autoregulation
5 Androgens

Page 42

40 Renal blood flow:
1 Is measured by para-amino hippuric acid clearance
2 Is autoregulated between mean arterial pressures of 80 and 180 mmHg
3 Equals one quarter of cardiac output
4 Goes mainly to the renal medulla
5 Is increased by high-dose (20 μg/kg/min) dopamine

Page 44

41 Hypokalaemia is caused by:
1 Diarrhoea
2 Frusemide therapy
3 Infusion of Hartmann's solution
4 Old age
5 Vomiting

42 Hypokalaemia is a feature of:
1 Acidosis
2 Cushing's syndrome
3 Conn's syndrome
4 Steroid therapy
5 Insulinoma

Page 45

43 Hyponatraemia causes:
1 Weakness
2 Headache
3 Vomiting
4 Peaked T waves on ECG
5 Positive Chvostek's sign

4 True
5 False

Renal blood flow:
1 True (fully cleared from plasma by kidneys)

2 True ~~other figures : 60 - 160~~ ↓(systolic press. 90 - 180 acc. to Whitehead)
3 True (about 1.2 l/min)
4 False (blood flow goes mainly to cortex)
5 False (decreased due to alpha stimulation)

Hypokalaemia is caused by:
1 True (loss of fluid containing K^+)
2 True (causes renal loss of K^+)
3 False (it contains potassium 3.5 mmol/l)
4 True (whole body K^+ depletion is common in old age)
5 True (gastric juice contains K^+)

Hypokalaemia is a feature of:
1 False (hypokalaemia is associated with alkalosis)
2 True
3 True
4 True
5 True

Hyponatraemia causes:
1 True
2 True
3 True
4 False (hyperkalaemia causes this)
5 False (hypocalcaemia causes this)

2 Pharmacology

Page 52
Phase 2 metabolism reactions:
1 May be impaired in the neonate
2 Conjugate isoprenaline with sulphate
3 Are used in the bromsulphthalein hepatic function test
4 Hydrolyse lignocaine
5 Are induced by cimetidine

Page 53
Pharmacokinetics:
1 In 1st order kinetics, decline is described by $-dC/dt = kC$
2 Rate constant k defines the fraction of drug eliminated in unit time
3 The half-life equals $0.693/k$
4 The volume of distribution of a drug is the amount of drug times the plasma concentration
5 Clearance by an organ equals blood flow times extraction ratio

Page 55
At receptors:
1 Agonists have occupancy and efficacy
2 Antagonists have occupancy and efficacy
3 Agonists have affinity and efficacy
4 Partial agonists have partial affinity
5 Occupancy fraction of receptors by a drug is defined by $[D]/(K_D + [D])$

Pharmacodynamics:
1 Efficacy is the maximum effect of an agonist
2 Potency is the minimum effect of an agonist
3 Down regulation is an increase in active receptor numbers
4 Potentiation is decreasing response to a drug stimulus
5 Tolerance is decreasing response to a drug stimulus

Phase 2 metabolism reactions:
1 True (due to hepatic immaturity)
2 True (conjugation with a radical is a typical phase 2 reaction)
3 True
4 False (hydrolysis is typically a phase 1 reaction)
5 False (inhibited by cimetidine)

Pharmacokinetics:
1 True

2 True
3 True

4 False (amount of drug divided by the plasma concentration)
5 True

At receptors:
1 True
2 False (occupancy but no efficacy)
3 True
4 False (they have partial efficacy)

5 True

Pharmacodynamics:
1 True
2 False (potency is dose required for a given effect)
3 False (decrease in active receptor numbers)
4 False (increasing response)
5 True

3 Physics

Page 57
Pressures:
1 1kg/sq cm = approximately 1 atmosphere
2 100 kPa = approximately 1 atmosphere
3 1 newton = the gravitational force of 1 kg
4 1 pascal = 1 newton per square metre
5 1 torr = 1 cm H_2O

Page 58
Boyle's law:
1 Relates pressure to temperature
2 Relates temperature to volume
3 Relates number of molecules to volume
4 Relates volume to absolute temperature
5 Relates pressure to volume

Page 59
Vapours:
1 Below the critical pressure, a gas cannot be liquefied

2 Below the critical temperature, a gas cannot be liquefied
3 Saturated vapour pressure increases linearly with temperature
4 Atmospheric pressure equals saturated vapour pressure at boiling point
5 Critical temperature of oxygen is $-119°C$

Osmotic pressure:
1 Osmolarity is the osmotic pressure per litre of solution
2 Osmolality is the osmotic pressure per kg of solvent
3 An aqueous solution of strength 1 osmol/l depresses freezing point by 1.86°C
4 Plasma osmolarity is about 290 mosmol/l
5 One milliosmole dissolved in 1 litre exerts an osmotic pressure of 22.4 atmospheres

Page 61
The following measure fluid flow:
1 Rotameter
2 Oscillometer
3 Respirometer
4 Glucometer
5 Ultrasound doppler

Pressures:
1 True
2 True
3 True
4 True
5 False (1 torr = 1 mmHg)

Boyle's law:
1 False (temperature is constant in Boyle's law)
2 False (temperature is constant in Boyle's law)
3 False (this is Avogadro's law)
4 False (this is Charles' law)
5 True

Vapours:
1 False (critical pressure is pressure needed to liquefy a gas at critical temperature)
2 False (above this temperature)
3 False (increases non-linearly)

4 True
5 True

Osmotic pressure:
1 True
2 True (similar to osmolarity in dilute aqueous solutions)

3 True
4 True (controlled by ADH)

5 False (1 osmole exerts this pressure)

The following measure fluid flow:
1 True (e.g. in anaesthetic machine) → gas, not fluid flow!
2 False (measures pressure, eg. blood pressure)
3 True (e.g. Wright's respirometer)
4 False (measures blood glucose)
5 True (e.g. noninvasive cardiac output monitoring, although primary measurement is of velocity)

Page 61
Heat:
1 1 calorie = 4.2 joules of energy
2 1 joule = 1 watt second
3 Latent heat is the temperature required to change unit mass of liquid to vapour
4 Specific heat is the energy required to warm 1 kg of a substance by 1°C
5 Thermal conductivity is the rate of heat transfer per unit area per unit temperature gradient

Page 62
Electricity:
1 A volt is the potential which releases 1 joule when 1 coulomb is transferred
2 A coulomb of electricity is transferred when 1 amp flows for 1 sec
3 Power consumption is 2.5 kW if 10 amps is flowing across a 250 V potential difference
4 Resistance equals potential difference divided by current
5 A watt of power equals a joule per second

Heat:
1 True
2 True

3 False (latent heat is the *energy* required)

4 True

5 True (high for copper, low for air)

Electricity:

1 True (the definition of voltage)

2 True

3 True (watts = amps × volts)
4 True (measured in ohms)
5 True (electric power is measured in watts)

4 Computing, clinical trials and statistics

Page 69
Clinical trials:
1 Null hypothesis states that there is a difference between two treatments
2 'Age and sex' matches controls completely
3 Statistical significance equals clinical significance
4 In a double-blind trial, observers and subjects are unaware of the treatments
5 Randomisation equals single blindness

Page 70
Statistics:
1 The mean is the observation which has half the observations above it and half below it
2 The mode is the most frequent observation
3 Standard deviation is the square root of the variance
4 Variance is the sum of the squares of the differences between observations and the mean, divided by their number
5 Standard error is the standard deviation (SD) divided by the number of observations

Page 71
Inferential tests:
1 Significant difference exists where 2 sample means differ by more than 2 of their standard errors of their difference
2 Chi-squared test cannot be used for small numbers of observations
3 Chi-squared equals the sum of the squares of the differences between the observed number and the expected number, divided by the expected number
4 A type 1 error is where the null hypothesis is wrongly accepted
5 A correlation coefficient of zero equals a significant relationship between two variables

Clinical trials:

1   False (no difference between the two)
2   False (match includes many other factors)
3   False ('there are lies, damned lies and ...')

4   True
5   False (a single blind trial merely means the subjects are
         unaware of the treatments)

Statistics:

1   False (this is the median)
2   True
3   True

4   True

5   False (SD divided by square root of the number)

Inferential tests:

1   True

2   True

3   True
4   False (where the null hypothesis is wrongly rejected)
5   False (a correlation coefficient of 1 or −1 is a perfect fit, zero
         indicates no relationship)

5 Preanaesthetic assessment and premedication

Page 80
Smoking causes:
1 Carboxyhaemoglobinaemia
2 Postoperative chest complications
3 Reduced ciliary activity
4 Reduced sputum
5 Reduced wound healing

When a patient is on regular clonidine medication:
1 Bronchoconstriction during anaesthesia is more likely to occur
2 It should be stopped before anaesthesia
3 The patient would require more premedication
4 Isoflurane is potentiated
5 Opioids are potentiated

Page 84
Monoamine oxidase inhibitors may:
1 Interact with pethidine to cause hypotension
2 Interact with fentanyl to cause coma
3 Interact with chlorpromazine to cause Cheyne–Stokes respiration
4 Interact with codeine to cause apnoea
5 Affect the body for 2 weeks after discontinuation

Page 91
Atropine:
1 Blocks nicotinic receptors
2 Causes auditory hyperacusis
3 Does not cross the blood brain barrier
4 Causes fetal tachycardia
5 Lasts longer in infants

Atropine:
1 Is a racemic mixture
2 Causes miosis
3 Is longer acting than glycopyrronium
4 Can cause arrhythmias
5 Stops neostigmine from raising intra-gut pressure

Page 92
Hyoscine:
1 Is a racemic mixture
2 Its central actions are reversed by neostigmine

3 Produces central excitation

Smoking causes:
1 True (impedes O_2 flux during anaesthesia)
2 True
3 True
4 False (increased sputum)
5 True (mechanism is obscure)

When a patient is on regular clonidine medication:
1 False
2 False (it reduces the stress response)
3 False (it potentiates analgesics and sedatives)
4 True (it potentiates the volatiles)
5 True (the patient requires less opioids)

Monoamine oxidase inhibitors may:
1 True   → hypertensicu !
2 True
3 False (chlorpromazine relieves these effects)
4 False (codeine can be used with confidence)
5 True

Atropine:
1 False (muscarinic)
2 True
3 False (it can cause central anticholinergic syndrome)
4 True (crosses placenta)
5 True (excretion is slower)

Atropine:
1 True (dextro- and laevorotatory)
2 False (mydriasis)
3 False (shorter acting)
4 True (large doses i.v. in young adults)
5 True (this inhibition is enhanced by volatile agents)

Hyoscine:
1 False (it is laevorotatory)
2 False (physostigmine needed as neostigmine does not
      cross the blood-brain barrier)
3 False (it is a good sedative)

4 Potentiates opiates
5 Is antiemetic

Page 93
Glycopyrronium:
1 Is a quarternary amine
2 Is shorter-acting than atropine
3 Causes fetal tachycardia
4 Crosses the blood-brain barrier
5 Is antiemetic

4 True
5 True (valuable in anaesthesia)

Glycopyrronium:
1 True
2 False (it lasts twice as long)
3 False (does not cross the placenta)
4 False
5 False

6 Anaesthetic equipment

Page 98
When full, anaesthetic gas cylinder pressures are:
1   137 bar for oxygen
2   137 bar for nitrous oxide
3   137 bar for carbon dioxide
4   137 bar for air
5   137 bar for entonox

Page 100
In the anaesthetic machine checklist recommended by the Association of Anaesthetists:
1   Bodok seals are subjected to a 'tug test'
2   It starts with all flowmeter valves closed
3   The audible oxygen failure alarm operates while the N_2O pressure is decreasing
4   The cylinder gauge pressure should hold up when the cylinder is turned off
5   Operation of the oxygen flush valve should decrease the pipeline pressure

Page 102
Rotameters:
1   Can have the control valve at either end of the tube
2   Must be vertical to be accurate
3   Depend on viscosity of gas at high flows
4   Depend on density of gas at low flows
5   The flow across the top of the rotameter tubes is from right to left

Page 104
The concentration delivered from a plenum vaporiser depends on:
1   Splitting ratio
2   Temperature of liquid
3   Vapour density
4   Saturated vapour pressure of liquid
5   The carrier gas

The pressure limiting valve on a 'Bain' gas circuit (system):
1   Opens at 4–8 kPa
2   Opens below the bursting pressure of the reservoir bag
3   Prevents all harm to the patient

4   Prevents pulmonary barotrauma
5   Works when the valve is screwed down tight

When full, anaesthetic gas cylinder pressures are:
1 True
2 False (54 bar)
3 False (50 bar)
4 True
5 True

In the anaesthetic machine checklist recommended by the Association of Anaesthetists:
1 False (Schrader valves are 'tug-tested')
2 False (open)

3 False (while oxygen pressure is decreasing)

4 False (it should fall) *depends on anaesthetic machine*

5 False (it should not change)

Rotameters:
1 True (some valves are distal to tube in USA)
2 True
3 False (depend on viscosity at low flow)
4 False (depend on density at high flow)

5 True (this reduces risk from O_2 leaks)

The concentration delivered from a plenum vaporiser depends on:
1 True (the control knob adjusts this)
2 True (various devices compensate for this)
3 False
4 True
5 False (no difference with commonly used gases)

The pressure limiting valve on a 'Bain' gas circuit (system):
1 True
2 True
3 False (pulmonary circulation obstructs before the
        valve opens [PA systolic pressure only 3.5 kPa])
4 True
5 True (designed to do this)

Page 107
Laryngeal masks:
1 Were invented by Brain
2 Protect the airway from regurgitation
3 Sit in the larynx
4 Size 4 cuff requires 4 ml of air
5 Require extension of the head for insertion

Page 110
Mapleson anaesthetic systems:
1 System M is the Magill system
2 The Lack system is system A
3 The Jackson Rees system is system D
4 The Bain system is system D
5 The minimum fresh gas flow in system E for spontaneous respiration is about twice the minute volume

Page 113
Soda lime:
1 Contains 5% $Ca(OH)_2$ and 90% $NaOH$
2 Horizontal cannister position prevents channelling
3 Occupies 95% of the space in the cannister
4 Heat of CO_2 absorption reaction decomposes sevoflurane
5 Soda lime powder is better than granules

Page 117
In adult mechanical ventilators:
1 Pressure support is where tidal volume is fixed
2 Volume control regulates respiratory rate
3 SIMV requires the patient to be paralysed
4 Inspiratory flow rate is less than 20 L/min.
5 VO_2 is calculated from CO_2 levels

The following increase peak inspiratory pressure during IPPV:
1 Closed system anaesthesia
2 Pneumothorax
3 Laparoscopic surgery
4 Cuff herniation
5 Salbutamol

Laryngeal masks:
1 True
2 False
3 False (they sit in the pharynx)
4 False (requires a maximum of 30 ml)
5 False (extension makes it easier, but they can be
        inserted without moving the neck)

Mapleson anaesthetic systems:
1 False (it is A)
2 True
3 False (it is F)
4 True

5 True   it's 2-3 times

Soda lime:
1 False (it is more than 90% Ca(OH)$_2$)
2 False (vertical position prevents this)
3 False (50%; the air space is needed for exhaled gas)
4 True
5 False (air space between granules lowers resistance
        to gas flow; powder might be inhaled)

In adult mechanical ventilators:
1 False (where inspiratory pressure is fixed)
2 True (indirectly, in many ventilators)
3 False (patient breathes spontaneously)
4 False (more than 60 L/min)
5 False (from inspired and expired O_2 and minute volume)

The following increase peak inspiratory pressure during IPPV:
1 False (no effect)
2 True (due to reduced compliance)
3 True (due to pressure on the diaphragm)
4 True (due to partial block of tracheal tube)
5 False (reduces it during bronchospasm)

Page 117

The following produce PEEP:

1 High frequency jet ventilation
2 Inspired : expired ratio of 2 to 1
3 Closed system anaesthesia
4 Double-lumen tubes
5 An expiratory pressure set at 10 cm water

Page 120

Sterilization:

1 Autoclaving destroys rubber and plastics
2 Boiling for 15 minutes destroys spores
3 Glutaraldehyde can destroy spores
4 Tubercle bacilli are destroyed by ethyl alcohol
5 Phenol destroys spores

The following produce PEEP:
1 True (the higher the frequency, the more the intrinsic PEEP)
2 False
3 False (no effect)
4 False (no effect)
5 True (this is 'extrinsic' PEEP)

Sterilization:
1 True
2 False (autoclaving needed)
3 True
4 False (they are alcohol-fast bacilli)
5 False

7 Inhalation anaesthesia

Page 128
Uptake of anaesthetic vapours in the lung depends on:
1 Cardiac output
2 Number of constituents in the inhaled mixture
3 Oil–water partition coefficient of the agent
4 Vapour concentration
5 Alveolar ventilation

Page 129
Minimum alveolar concentration of an anaesthetic agent:
1 Is the concentration producing lack of reflex response to skin incision in 95% of patients
2 MAC fractions of agents in mixtures are additive
3 MAC of desflurane is 6%
4 MAC of sevoflurane is 2%
5 Must be measured at sea-level

Page 132
The 'quadrant of anaesthesia' includes:
1 Suppression of reflexes
2 Suppression of stress response
3 Relaxation of smooth muscle
4 Narcosis
5 Relaxation of skeletal muscle

Nitrous oxide:
1 Was discovered in 1772 by J. Priestley
2 Was used as anaesthetic by Colton in 1844
3 Is used to treat septic shock syndrome
4 Cylinder contents are measured by pressure gauge
5 Has a critical temperature of 36.5°C

Nitrous oxide:
1 Boils at minus 89°C
2 Has a blood–gas partition coefficient of 0.47
3 Is organic
4 Has a brain–blood partition coefficient of 1
5 Reversal by naloxone has been described

Uptake of anaesthetic vapours in the lung depends on:
1 True (a low cardiac output reduces uptake)
2 True (second gas effect speeds uptake)
3 False (blood–gas partition coefficient)
4 True
5 True (important in clinical anaesthesia)

Minimum alveolar concentration of an anaesthetic agent:

1 False (lack of response in 50% of patients)
2 True
3 True
4 True
5 True (minimum alveolar partial pressure is a more versatile
        measure)

The 'quadrant of anaesthesia' includes:
1 True
2 True
3 False
4 True
5 True

Nitrous oxide:
1 True
2 True
3 False (nitric oxide has been used)
4 False (measured by weighing)
5 True

Nitrous oxide:
1 True
2 True (it is rather insoluble)
3 False (it is an inorganic chemical)
4 True (thus affects the brain rapidly on induction)
5 True

Page 138
Halothane:
1 Is 2,bromo-2,chloro-trifluoro-ethane
2 Rubber–gas partition coefficient is 120 at 20°C

3 SVP is 243 mmHg at 20°C
4 Is a good analgesic
5 Relaxes smooth muscle

Halothane:
1 Is metabolised by reduction
2 Is metabolised by oxidation
3 Constricts the uterus
4 Relaxes trismus
5 Produces tachypnoea

Page 141
Enflurane:
1 Is an alkane
2 SVP is 175 mmHg at 20°C
3 Depresses the myocardium
4 Vasodilates
5 Is metabolised to bromide

Page 143
Isoflurane:
1 Is a methyl ethyl ether
2 Depresses muscle tone
3 Depresses respiration
4 Causes tachypnoea
5 Dilates coronary arteries

Isoflurane:
1 Flattens the EEG at 2 MAC
2 0.2% of the drug is metabolised in the body
3 Does not affect the pregnant uterus
4 Does not react with soda lime
5 Antagonises nondepolarising relaxants

Isoflurane:
1 Usually causes hypertension
2 Can cause tachycardia
3 Is a dose-dependent cerebral vasodilator
4 Raises intraocular pressure
5 Can cause coronary steal

Halothane:
1 True
2 True (i.e. it dissolves in the rubber components of anaesthetic machines)
3 True (similar to isoflurane)
4 False
5 True

Halothane:
1 True
2 True
3 False (relaxes the uterus)
4 True (a very useful clinical effect)
5 True (can be masked by opioids)

Enflurane:
1 False (an ether; trifluoro-chloroethyl difluoro-methyl ether)
2 True
3 True (tends to produce hypotension)
4 True (tends to produce hypotension)
5 False (metabolised to fluoride)

Isoflurane:
1 True (and a fluorinated drug)
2 True (a clinically useful feature)
3 True
4 True
5 True (normally a useful feature)

Isoflurane:
1 True
2 True
3 False (more than 1 MAC relaxes it)
4 True
5 False (potentiates)

Isoflurane:
1 False (usually causes slight hypotension)
2 True
3 True
4 False (tends to lower it)
5 True (in rare cases of distal coronary occlusion)

Page 145
Desflurane:
1 Boils at room temperature
2 Blood–gas partition coefficient is less than N_2O
3 Has a MAC of 6%
4 Requires refrigerated vaporisers
5 Reacts with soda lime

Page 146
Sevoflurane:
1 Reacts with soda lime
2 Metabolites are completely harmless

3 MAC is 6%
4 Is chemically an alkane
5 Blood–gas partition coefficient is 0.6

Desflurane:
1 True (boiling point is 23.5°C)
2 True (coefficient is 0.4)
3 True
4 False (heated vaporisers currently in use) *pressurized!*
5 False (it is stable with soda lime)

Sevoflurane:
1 True (20% degradation)
2 False (nephrotoxic fluoride levels and compound A have been
    seen after prolonged exposure)
3 False (MAC is 2%)
4 False (a fluorinated methyl isopropyl ether)
5 True

8 Gases used in association with anaesthesia

Page 151
Oxygen:
1 Is, semantically, an acid producer
2 Critical pressure is 50.8 bar
3 Boiling point is $-183°C$
4 Is absorbed on to zeolites
5 Molecular weight is 16

Page 152
Carbon dioxide:
1 Is the main stimulant of the respiratory centre
2 Used as an anaesthetic by Henry Hill Hickman

3 Molecular weight is 44
4 Critical temperature is $-31°C$
5 Cylinder pressure is 137 bar

Carbon dioxide:
1 Expired concentration is 4%
2 Alveolar concentration is 50%
3 Stored as liquid in cylinders
4 Causes catecholamine release from adrenals
5 Room air contains 3%

Page 155
Helium:
1 Gives a lower Reynolds number than oxygen
2 Is lighter than hydrogen
3 Similar viscosity to oxygen
4 Very soluble in water
5 21% O_2/79% helium mixture has a S.G. of a third that of air

Oxygen:
1 True (oxy = acid; gen = producer)
2 True
3 True
4 False (N_2 is absorbed in oxygen concentrators)
5 False (atomic weight is 16)

Carbon dioxide:
1 True
2 True (commemorated in the Hickman Medal of the Royal Society of Medicine)
3 True (same as nitrous oxide)
4 False (31°C)
5 False (50 bar)

Carbon dioxide:
1 True
2 False (5%)
3 True
4 True
5 False (0.03%)

Helium:
1 True
2 False (2nd lightest gas; density 0.17 kg/cu.m)
3 True
4 False (0.0088ml/ml; used for lung volume estimation)
5 True (may be useful in upper airway obstruction)

9 Intravenous anaesthetic agents

Page 160
Thiopentone:
1 pH of 2.5% solution is 10.5
2 Increases cerebral oxygen consumption
3 Sodium carbonate is present in thiopentone ampoule
4 Is analgesic
5 Increases pulmonary vascular resistance

Thiopentone:
1 Stimulates secretion of ADH
2 Increases intraocular tension
3 Produces retrograde amnesia
4 Its elimination half-life is about 9 hours
5 Is indicated in dystrophia myotonica

Page 161
Arterial toxicity of thiopentone:
1 Is due to acidity of the drug
2 Occurs because of lack of dilution of the drug in the arterial tree
3 Involves crystallisation of haemoglobin
4 Causes pain
5 Treated by intra-arterial heparin

Page 168
Etomidate:
1 Is dissolved in 35% aqueous propylene glycol
2 Does not lower arterial pressure
3 Is antiemetic
4 Dissolves in erythrocytes
5 Causes cortisol secretion

Page 170
Propofol:
1 Has no active metabolites
2 Causes alkalosis
3 Has quicker recovery than methohexitone
4 Has an effective blood concentration of 34 micrograms per ml
5 May cause green coloration of urine with prolonged use

Propofol:
1 Is di-iso-propyl-phenol
2 Is antiemetic

Thiopentone:
1 True (strongly alkaline)
2 False (decreases it, and may protect the brain)
3 True (prevents free acid formation by atmospheric CO_2)
4 False (it is antanalgesic)
5 False (decreases it)

Thiopentone:
1 True (causes oliguria during anaesthesia)
2 False (decreases it)
3 True (a clinically useful effect)
4 True
5 False (very small doses cause prolonged apnoea)

Arterial toxicity of thiopentone:
1 False (due to its alkalinity)
2 True
3 True
4 True (the first clinical sign)
5 True (the acidity of heparin reverses the alkalinity of thiopentone)

Etomidate:
1 True
2 True
3 False (commonly causes nausea)
4 True
5 False (it suppresses cortisol and is contraindicated for sedation in intensive care)

Propofol:
1 True
2 False
3 True (but the difference is small)
4 False (about 3.4 μg/ml)
5 True (due to phenol excretion)

Propofol:
1 True
2 True

3 Is a vasoconstrictor
4 Potentiates and prolongs alfentanil
5 Is safe in dystrophia myotonica

Page 173
Diazepam:
1 Is water soluble
2 Is inhibited by cimetidine
3 Acts via GABA chloride channels
4 Increases serum potassium
5 Potentiates intravenous induction agents

Page 174
Midazolam:
1 Produces anterograde amnesia
2 Is water soluble
3 Is a respiratory depressant
4 Excretion half-life is 14.5 hr
5 Does not cause upper airway obstruction

Page 175
Fentanyl:
1 Is highly lipophobic
2 Is excreted in bile
3 Is absorbed from the intestine
4 Causes tachycardia
5 Causes muscular rigidity

Page 176
Alfentanil:
1 Is more rapidly metabolised in children
2 Is antiemetic
3 Causes bradycardia
4 Is a smooth muscle stimulant
5 Is a respiratory stimulant

Alfentanil:
1 Is more lipid soluble than fentanyl
2 Has a higher volume of distribution than fentanyl
3 Has a longer terminal half-life than lofentanyl
4 Is more potent than sufentanil
5 Has its terminal half-life prolonged by propofol

3 False (vasodilator which causes hypotension)
4 True
5 True (but myoclonic effects are prolonged)

Diazepam:
1 False (dissolved in propylene glycol or soya emulsion)
2 False (it is potentiated)
3 True
4 False (decreases it)
5 True

Midazolam:
1 True
2 True
3 True
4 False (about 1.45 hr)
5 False

Fentanyl:
1 False (lipophilic)
2 True
3 True (enterohepatic recirculation)
4 False (bradycardia)
5 True (especially of the body wall)

Alfentanil:
1 True ($T_{1/2}$ 63 min compared with 95 min in adults)
2 False (a nauseating drug)
3 True
4 True
5 False (it is a respiratory depressant)

Alfentanil:
1 False
2 False (much smaller)
3 False (lofentanyl lasts for many hours)
4 False
5 True

Page 758
Diamorphine:
1 Is more lipid soluble than morphine
2 Is more rapidly hydrolysed than morphine
3 Causes hypotonicity of the small intestine
4 Is metabolised to morphine
5 Is more potent than morphine

Page 179
Ketamine:
1 Its chronotropic effect is blocked by verapamil
2 Its inotropic effect is blocked by verapamil
3 Increases plasma noradrenaline
4 Is a bronchoconstrictor
5 Inhibits salivation

Ketamine:
1 Is a pulmonary vasoconstrictor
2 Is analgesic
3 Is antiemetic
4 Light ketamine anaesthesia maintains upper airway reflexes
5 The unpleasant dreams on emergence are more common in children

Page 182
Total intravenous anaesthesia:
1 Does not require resuscitation equipment
2 Can be monitored by oesophageal contractions
3 Initial infusion rate of propofol 1% in ml/hr equals body weight in kg
4 The airway is secure
5 Oxygen is not required

Diamorphine:
1 True
2 True
3 True
4 True
5 True (about 1.5 times more potent)

Ketamine:
1 False
2 True
3 True
4 False (it is a bronchodilator)
5 False (causes salivation and may need atropine cover)

Ketamine:
1 True
2 True (its main clinical use)
3 False (may cause nausea)
4 True

5 False

Total intravenous anaesthesia:
1 False (full resuscitation equipment is needed)
2 True (less than 4/min suggests adequate anaesthesia)

3 True
4 False (needs to be constantly monitored)
5 False (added O_2 frequently needed)

10 Muscle relaxants

Page 190
The skeletal neuromuscular junction:
1 MEPPs are caused by adrenaline release
2 The ACh receptor is a lipid molecule
3 The resting end plate potential is 70 mV
4 Is blocked by penicillins
5 Is blocked by dantrolene

Page 192
Non-depolarising relaxants:
1 Potentiated by Mg^{++}
2 Normally potentiated by suxamethonium
3 Normally potentiated by acidosis
4 Normally potentiated by isoflurane
5 Normally potentiated by neostigmine

Page 193
Depolarising relaxants:
1 Cause fade
2 Cause fasciculation
3 Are antagonised by halothane
4 Are one of the causes of malignant hyperpyrexia
5 Are antagonised by magnesium

The transcutaneous nerve stimulator for monitoring the neuromuscular junction:
1 Frequency for the train of four is 2 Hz
2 T_4/T_1 ratio of 15% shows adequate relaxation for laparotomy
3 Train of four (TOF) count of 1 to 2 should be adequate relaxation for laparotomy
4 Post-tetanic count (PTC) of 15 shows adequate relaxation for laparotomy
5 Double-burst stimulation is used for assessing slight block

Page 198
The following are differential diagnoses of incomplete reversal of relaxant:
1 Hypothermia
2 Addisonian crisis
3 Cretinism
4 Botulism
5 Hypocalcaemia

The skeletal neuromuscular junction:
1 False (caused by acetylcholine release)
2 False (protein molecule)
3 False (-70 mV)
4 False (blocked to some extent by aminoglycosides)
5 False (dantrolene blocks the sarcoplasmic Ca^{++}
      release channel: the ryanodine receptor)

Non-depolarising relaxants:
1 True
2 False (most of them are antagonised)
3 True (and prolonged)   *But not atracurium!*
4 True
5 False (reversed by neostigmine)

Depolarising relaxants:
1 False (this is caused by non-depolarising relaxants)
2 True
3 True
4 True
5 False (potentiated by Mg^{++})

The transcutaneous nerve stimulator for monitoring the neuromuscular junction:
1 True
2 True

3 True

4 False (PTC count of 1–5 is adequate for laparotomy)
5 True (bursts separated by 750 ms)

The following are differential diagnoses of incomplete reversal of relaxant:
1 True
2 True
3 False
4 True
5 False (hypocalcaemia causes muscle spasms of tetany)

Page 199
Atracurium:
1 Is metabolised to laudanum
2 Is not absorbed from i.m. injection
3 Is an antihistamine
4 Is shorter acting in hypothermia
5 Relaxes the fetus

Atracurium:
1 Is metabolised by the liver
2 Is excreted by the kidney
3 Has a vagolytic side effect
4 Its histamine release is a result of C_3 conversion
5 Laudanosine has a half-life of 23 min

Page 200
Vecuronium:
1 Dose is best estimated from body weight
2 Potentiated by previous suxamethonium
3 Releases histamine
4 Chemically derived from tubocurarine
5 The tertiary N at 2beta in the A ring gives shorter duration than pancuronium

Page 202
Mivacurium:
1 Is a steroid
2 Is metabolised in the liver
3 Has a duration of 30 min
4 Onset in 30 sec
5 Is vagolytic

Pipecuronium:
1 Is a steroid
2 Has a duration of 30 min
3 Relaxing dose is 0.05 mg/kg
4 Relies on renal excretion
5 Is potentiated by enflurane

Page 203
Neostigmine:
1 Prevents hydrolysis of acetylcholine
2 Is broken down by serum cholinesterase
3 Is excreted by the kidneys

Atracurium:
1 False (laudanosine is one of its metabolites)
2 False
3 False (releases histamine and may cause bronchospasm)
4 False (length doubled at 25°C)
5 False (does not cross the placenta)

Atracurium:
1 False (by alkaline hydrolysis in plasma)
2 False (alkaline hydrolysis in plasma)
3 False (no direct effect on heart rate)
4 False
5 False (234 min, i.e. long-acting)

Vecuronium:
1 False (0.1 mg × *lean* body mass)
2 True
3 False
4 False (derived from pancuronium)

5 True

Mivacurium:
1 False (a benzylisoquinolinium)
2 False (by plasma cholinesterase)
3 False (10–15 min)
4 False (1.5–3.5 min)
5 False (slight bradycardia sometimes seen)

Pipecuronium:
1 True
2 False (1–2 hr)
3 True
4 True (care needed in renal failure)
5 True

Neostigmine:
1 True
2 True (and it inhibits cholinesterase)
3 True

4 Is a nicotinic stimulator
5 Is a muscarinic antagonist

Page 205
Suxamethonium:
1 Is a quarternary ammonium compound
2 Is required in higher doses in infants
3 Is vagolytic
4 Onset in 90 sec
5 Hydrolysed by 2nd order pharmacokinetics

Page 207
Plasma cholinesterase deficiency may be seen:
1 In malnutrition
2 In pregnancy
3 In inheritance of the silent gene
4 In neonates
5 In hepatic failure

Page 208
Postoperative apnoea may be caused by:
1 Hypocapnia
2 Stimulation of pulmonary stretch receptors
3 Succinyl monocholine
4 Sufentanyl
5 Metabolic acidosis

Suxamethonium causes:
1 Lowered intraocular pressure
2 Muscle pains more frequently in adult women
3 Muscle pains more frequently in pregnancy
4 Relaxation in patients with dystrophia myotonica
5 Anaphylaxis

4 True
5 False (muscarinic stimulator)

Suxamethonium:
1 True
2 True (2 mg/kg)
3 False (slows the heart)
4 False (one circulation time)
5 False (hydrolysis is 1st order pharmacokinetics)

Plasma cholinesterase deficiency may be seen:
1 True
2 True (but rarely clinically significant)
3 True
4 True
5 True

Postoperative apnoea may be caused by:
1 True
2 False (depression of these)
3 True (a metabolite of suxamethonium)
4 True (opioid effect on respiratory centre)
5 True (depression of neuromuscular function) *must be pretty severe to do so*

Suxamethonium causes:
1 False (raised IOP)
2 True
3 False (less frequently in pregnancy)
4 False (causes rigidity in this disease)
5 True (rarely)

11 Tracheal intubation

Page 220
The cuff of a tracheal tube:
1 Deflates with time
2 Intracuff pressure should not exceed 100 mmHg
3 Prevents aspiration of pharyngeal contents into the lungs
4 Its filling tube has a longer intramural length in a nasal tube
5 Causes a fall of IPPV pressure when herniated

Page 230
Rapid absorption of the following drugs occurs after endotracheal administration:
1 Adrenaline
2 Thiopentone
3 Lignocaine
4 Naloxone
5 Atropine

Page 234
When intubating children:
1 The epiglottis is shorter and flatter than in adults
2 The narrowest part of the upper airway is the cricoid
3 Length of trachea is age divided by 4, plus 4 cm
4 The rima glottidis is level with C3/4
5 The RAE tube cannot enter the right main bronchus

The cuff of a tracheal tube:
1 False (inflates due to N_2O absorption)
2 False (not exceed 22 mmHg, the capillary perfusion pressure)
3 True
4 True (to avoid nasal trauma)
5 False (a rise due to obstruction of tube)

Rapid absorption of the following drugs occurs after endotracheal administration:
1 True
2 False (but true for diazepam)
3 True
4 True
5 True

When intubating children:
1 False (longer and more curved)
2 True (there should be a leak around the tube)
3 True *wrong, that's the formula for calculating internal diameter*
4 True (higher than in adults)
5 False (it may do; and has a Murphy eye to prevent
        upper bronchus blockage)

12 Artificial ventilation of the lungs

Page 240
Intrapleural pressure is:
1 About 100 cm H_2O during a cough
2 Greater at the base than the apex in erect posture
3 -10 cm H_2O during a spontaneous inspiration
4 Decreased by IPPV
5 Greater in adults than children

IPPV causes:
1 Respiratory acidosis
2 Increase of deadspace
3 Potentiation of thoracic pump
4 Increase of body water
5 Increase of CVP

Page 241
PEEP:
1 Reduces cardiac output
2 Reduces deadspace
3 Reduces FRC
4 Reduces intracranial pressure
5 Reduces urine flow

Page 244
The ideal ventilator:
1 Has a maximum inspiratory flow rate of 8 l/min
2 Is easy to sterilise
3 Adapts for children
4 Has facilities for PEEP and SIMV
5 Is usable in closed systems

Intrapleural pressure is:
1 True
2 True (because of the weight of the lungs)
3 True
4 False (increased)
5 False

IPPV causes:
1 False (respiratory alkalosis usually)
2 True
3 False (abolition of thoracic pump)
4 True (over a period of days)
5 True

PEEP:
1 True (by impeding venous return)
2 False (increases deadspace by dilating airways) .
3 False (increases FRC by opening alveoli)
4 False (increases ICP by impeding venous return)
5 True (increases ADH secretion)

The ideal ventilator:
1 False (80 l/min)
2 True
3 True
4 True
5 True

13 Production of ischaemia during operations

Page 248
Bleeding during surgery:
1 Is reduced by elevating the operative site
2 Is reduced by local vasopressin
3 Is reduced by bradycardia
4 Is reduced by hypertension
5 Is reduced by hypocapnia

Pages 252–3
Glyceryl trinitrate in clinical doses:
1 Reduces preload
2 Reduces afterload
3 Reduces intracranial pressure
4 Reduces intraocular pressure
5 Reduces intracranial blood volume

Bleeding during surgery:
1 True (reduces venous ooze)
2 True (capillary constrictor)
3 True (reduces arterial bleeding)
4 False (reduced by hypotension)
5 True (via vasoconstriction and reduced cardiac output)

Glyceryl trinitrate in clinical doses:
1 True
2 True
3 True
4 True
5 False

14 Accidents, complications and sequelae of anaesthesia

Page 262
Upper airway obstruction:
1 Stridor implies that the adult airway is reduced to less than 6 mm diameter
2 May be caused by the epiglottis
3 Is solved by the use of a laryngeal mask
4 Is solved by using a relaxant
5 Causes paradoxical respiration

Page 264
Postoperative pulmonary atelectasis is characterised by:
1 CO_2 retention
2 Bradypnoea
3 Bradycardia
4 Chest pain
5 Increased radiolucency on chest X-ray

Page 266
Postoperative hypoxia is made worse by:
1 Upper airway obstruction
2 Smoking
3 Obesity
4 Advancing age
5 Sleep apnoea syndrome

Page 267
Pulmonary embolism (PE):
1 May be caused by hypernephroma
2 May be caused by liquor amnii
3 Is more likely in smokers
4 Is more likely in the obese
5 Is more likely in pleurisy

Page 269
Gas embolism can result from:
1 Cardiac surgery
2 CVP lines
3 Hydrogen peroxide irrigation of body cavities
4 Laparoscopic surgery
5 Blood warming coils

Upper airway obstruction:

1 True
2 True (especially a large floppy one)
3 False (obstruction is often at or below the larynx)
4 False (only if due to laryngeal spasm)
5 True (chest and abdomen move in a 'see-saw' way)

Postoperative pulmonary atelectasis is characterised by:
1 False (by hypoxia)
2 False (tachypnoea)
3 False (tachycardia)
4 True (often at the site of atelectasis)
5 False (decreased radiolucency at the site of atelectasis)

Postoperative hypoxia is made worse by:
1 True
2 True (partly due to carboxyhaemoglobinaemia)
3 True (due to alveolar and airways closure)
4 True (due to impaired lung function)
5 True (worst in the first 2 to 3 postoperative nights)

Pulmonary embolism (PE):
1 True (the tumour itself may embolise)
2 True (amniotic fluid embolus in obstetric practice)
3 True (increased risk of DVT)
4 True (increased risk of DVT)
5 False (but pleurisy may result from PE)

Gas embolism can result from:
1 True
2 True
3 True
4 True (from compressed CO_2 in the abdomen)
5 True (if not pre-filled with solution)

Page 271

During anaesthesia in the prone position:
1 Breathing is easier
2 Blindness may occur
3 Regurgitation of stomach contents is facilitated
4 Neuropraxia is a risk
5 Malignant hyperpyrexia is more likely to occur

Page 280

Unplanned awareness in general anaesthesia may produce:
1 Increased spectral edge frequencies
2 More than 10 lower oesophageal contractions per minute
3 Shorter latencies in somatosensory evoked potentials
4 Unexplained tachycardia
5 Unexplained increase in relaxation

Page 282

Unplanned awareness in general anaesthesia may be reduced by:
1 Diazepam
2 Hyoscine
3 Atropine
4 Ear muffs
5 Thiopentone

Page 284

Malignant hyperpyrexia:
1 The abnormality originates in the sarcoplasmic reticulum
2 Is associated with the use of suxamethonium
3 Is associated with the use of procaine
4 Causes extracellular calcium release
5 Its severity is related to the dose of the trigger agent

Page 286

At a body temperature of 30°C:
1 Cerebral oxygen consumption is about 40% of normal
2 Arrhythmias occur
3 Tachycardia is seen
4 Alkalosis may occur due to increased solubility of CO_2
5 Blood viscosity is reduced

Page 289

The following should be part of your immediate management of anaphylaxis:
1 Adrenaline

During anaesthesia in the prone position:
1 False (IPPV often used)
2 True (from pressure on retina)
3 True (the airway may need to be protected)
4 True (from pressure on superficial nerves)
5 False

Unplanned awareness in general anaesthesia may produce:
1 False (reduced spectral edge frequencies)
2 True (easy to measure, but unreliable)
3 True
4 True
5 False (no effect)

Unplanned awareness in general anaesthesia may be reduced by:
1 True (it produces anterograde amnesia)
2 True (it produces anterograde amnesia)
3 False (it causes auditory hyperacusis)
4 True (most awareness is auditory)
5 True (it may produce retrograde amnesia)

Malignant hyperpyrexia:
1 True (at the ryanodine receptor)
2 True
3 False (procaine is safe)
4 False (intracellular calcium release)
5 True

At a body temperature of 30°C:
1 True
2 True (a considerable risk of VF)
3 False (bradycardia is usually seen)
4 True
5 False (it is increased)

The following should be part of your immediate management of anaphylaxis:
1 True

2 Intravenous colloids
3 Oxygen
4 Steroids
5 Antihistamines

Page 292
Hepatitis B transmission:
1 Occurs through close physical contact
2 Occurs via most body fluids
3 Simple infectious carriers have anti-HB e Ag
4 Fomites can be sterilised by 3 hr in hypochlorite or glutaraldehyde
5 Seroconversion over 100 i.u. per ml is the sign of effective immunisation

2 True
3 True
4 True (less urgent than 1, 2 and 3)
5 True (less urgent than 1, 2 and 3)

Hepatitis B transmission:
1 True
2 True
3 True

4 True

5 True

15 Drugs used in association with anaesthesia

Page 300
Adrenergic receptors:
1 Are beta-1 in the heart
2 Are beta-2 in the bronchi
3 Vasoconstriction is usually via alpha receptors
4 Hepatic glycogenolysis is via beta-1 receptors
5 Reduction of gut motility is via alpha receptors

Page 301
Adrenaline:
1 Is a pure alpha agonist
2 Shortens coagulation time
3 Decreases platelet stickiness
4 Its initial adult dose in ACLS is 1 mg
5 Its initial dose in anaphylaxis is 1 mg

Adrenaline secretion is caused by:
1 Parasympathetic stimulation
2 Clonidine
3 Carbon dioxide
4 Cardiac arrest
5 Hypoxia

Stimulation of alpha receptors causes:
1 Platelet aggregation
2 Coronary vasoconstriction
3 Some pilomotor contraction
4 Systemic venoconstriction
5 Miosis

Page 302
Noradrenaline:
1 Is an alpha agonist
2 May be used to raise the systemic vascular resistance in septic shock
3 Is the main sympathetic neurotransmitter
4 Infusion dose is $1–20 \mu g/min$
5 Is the vasoconstrictor of choice with local analgesics

Page 304
Methoxamine:
1 Is a vasodilator
2 Lasts for 10 min
3 Stimulates the heart

Adrenergic receptors:
1 True (blocked by e.g. atenolol)
2 True (stimulated by salbutamol)
3 True (blocked by phentolamine)
4 True
5 True

Adrenaline:
1 False (alpha and beta)
2 True (part of fear fight and flight response)
3 False (increases it)
4 True
5 False (0.1 mg)

Adrenaline secretion is caused by:
1 False (adrenals have sympathetic supply)
2 False (clonidine reduces central sympathetic drive)
3 True (reflex effect on adrenals)
4 True
5 True (reflex effect on adrenals)

Stimulation of alpha receptors causes:
1 True
2 True (direct effect)
3 True
4 True
5 False (causes mydriasis)

Noradrenaline:
1 True

2 True
3 True
4 True
5 False (may cause severe hypertension)

Methoxamine:
1 False (it is a pure vasoconstrictor)
2 False (lasts for 1 hr)
3 False (no direct effect)

4 Causes desire to void urine
5 Causes bradycardia

Page 304
Felypressin:
1 Is mainly an antidiuretic drug
2 Has no effect on cardiac rhythm
3 Causes secondary vasodilatation
4 Has no reaction with monoamine oxidase inhibitors
5 Dilates the coronary arteries

Page 305
Dopamine:
1 A dose of 2 μg/kg/min stimulates D receptors
2 A dose of 5 μg/kg/min stimulates beta receptors
3 A dose of 20 μg/kg/min stimulates alpha receptors
4 A dose of 2 μg/kg/min augments gut wall perfusion
5 Does not occur naturally in the body

Page 306
Isoprenaline:
1 Has positive inotropic cardiac effects
2 Has positive chronotropic cardiac effects
3 Increases skeletal muscle perfusion
4 Weakens skeletal muscle performance
5 Constricts bronchi

Page 309
Non-selective beta blockers:
1 Relieve asthma
2 May cause cardiac failure
3 May cause hypoglycaemia in diabetics
4 May aggravate Raynaud's phenomenon
5 Reduce reflex responses to haemorrhage

Page 311
Nifedipine:
1 Has a slow onset
2 Is a coronary vasodilator
3 Is used in Prinzmetal's angina
4 Can produce atrioventricular blockade
5 Is indicated in hypotension

4 True
5 True (due to baroreceptor reflex)

Felypressin:
1 False (it has little or no antidiuretic effect)
2 True
3 False (unlike adrenaline)
4 True (unlike adrenaline)
5 False (constricts them)

Dopamine:
1 True (in the renal blood vessels)
2 True (in the heart)
3 True (giving vasoconstriction)
4 True (may help prevent endotoxinaemia)
5 False

Isoprenaline:
1 True
2 True
3 True
4 True (only a problem for athletes)
5 False (dilates bronchi)

Non-selective beta blockers:
1 False (cause bronchospasm)
2 True (where cardiac contractility is critical)
3 True
4 True
5 True (important in anaesthesia and trauma)

Nifedipine:
1 False (its rapid onset is very useful)
2 True (valuable in coronary disease)
3 True
4 False (verapamil does this)
5 False (in hypertension)

Page 311
Nifedipine:
1 Is stopped a week before coronary artery surgery
2 Is antagonised by volatile anaesthetics
3 Decreases MAC values of volatile anaesthetics
4 A typical dose is 100 mg
5 Antagonises non-depolarising muscle relaxants

Page 313
Heparin:
1 Is reversed by prostanol
2 Has a half-life of 1 hr
3 Hydrolysed by hepatic heparinase
4 Excreted in urine
5 Extracorporeal circuit dose is 30 units/kg

Prothrombin time (or INR) can be helpful in the diagnosis of:
1 Scurvy

2 Disseminated intravascular coagulation
3 Haemophilia
4 Thrombocytopenic purpura
5 Warfarin therapy

These results indicate adequate anticoagulation against venous thrombosis:
1 Prothrombin time of 10 sec; control of 14.5 sec
2 APTT of 32 sec; control of 25 sec
3 International Normalised Ratio of 0.5
4 Bleeding time of 3–5 min
5 ACT of 100 sec

Nifedipine:
1 False (it is usually continued)
2 False (potentiated)
3 True
4 False (10 mg)
5 False (potentiates them)

Heparin:
1 False (protamine, 1 mg/100 units remaining heparin)
2 True (enables calculation of remaining drug)
3 True
4 True
5 False (300 units/kg)

Prothrombin time (or INR) can be helpful in the diagnosis of:
1 False (scurvy is vitamin C deficiency, the capillaries are abnormal)
2 True
3 False
4 False (this is a platelet deficiency)
5 True (the normal measurement for control)

These results indicate adequate anticoagulation against venous thrombosis:
1 False (PT ratio should be about 2)
2 False (APTT ratio should be about 2)
3 False (INR should be about 2)
4 False (this is normal and anyway is not a useful guide)
5 False (not used for this purpose)

16 Immediate postoperative care

Page 318
The patient who becomes cyanosed in the postoperative recovery ward:
1   May need laying on his side
2   May be hypervolaemic
3   May need sitting up
4   Will always need oxygen
5   May need neostigmine

The patient who becomes hypotensive in the postoperative recovery ward:
1   May be hypovolaemic
2   May need antibiotics

3   Will always need oxygen
4   May need an opiate
5   May need an ECG recording

Page 319
The high dependency unit:
1   Is equipped with specialised monitoring
2   IPPV may be given for several days
3   Is a safe location for the use of extradural opiates
4   Is for surgical patients only
5   Has a nurse/patient ratio of 1 to 5

The patient who becomes cyanosed in the postoperative recovery ward:
1   True (airway obstruction is the commonest cause)
2   True (causing pulmonary oedema)
3   True (the patient with respiratory failure often benefits)
4   True (and adequate ventilation)
5   True (inadequate reversal is a common problem)

The patient who becomes hypotensive in the postoperative recovery ward:
1   True (the classic tachycardia and restlessness are often absent)
2   True (bacteraemia, after e.g. urology procedures, causes hypotension)
3   True (and adequate ventilation)
4   True (pain can cause hypotension)
5   True (silent myocardial infarcts cause hypotension)

The high dependency unit:
1   True
2   False (no more than a few hours)
3   True
4   False
5   False (1 nurse to 2 patients is more usual)

17 Intravascular techniques, infusion and blood transfusion

Pages 324–326
Intravenous fluids:
1 Most crystalloid solutions are less acidic than plasma
2 Dextrans are carbohydrate polymers produced by *Leuconostoc mesenteroides*
3 Gelatins are largely excreted by the kidneys
4 Substituted starch solutions have a higher incidence of adverse reactions than the gelatins
5 The degree of substitution of a starch refers to the fraction of glucose units with hydroxyethyl moieties

Blood substitutes:
1 Haemoglobin in free solution has a low P_{50}
2 Pyridoxal-5-phosphate can be used as a substitute for 2,3-DPG to correct the P_{50} of haemoglobin solutions
3 Red cell stroma is nephrotoxic
4 Fluorocarbons are soluble in blood
5 Fluorocarbon blood substitutes have linear dissociation curves for all gases

Page 329
Blood donors in the UK are screened for antibodies to:
1 HIV-2
2 Treponema pallidum
3 Hepatitis A
4 Hepatitis C
5 Brucella

Page 330
Blood storage for 2 weeks at 4–6°C:
1 Destroys half of the factor V
2 Destroys well over half the factor VIII
3 Leaves the platelets functioning adequately
4 Has little effect on factor VII
5 Is not possible if red cells are suspended in SAGM

Blood transfusion:
1 The addition of adenine to CPD blood helps to preserve red cell ATP
2 Nearly one-eighth of a bag of CPD whole blood is the CPD solution
3 Blood should not be returned to its refrigerator if it has been out of it for over ½ hour
4 ABO antibodies are present in a neonate

Intravenous fluids:
1 False (most have a low pH)

2 True (molecular weights indicated by '40', '70')
3 True

4 False (the converse is true)

5 True (often about 50–70%)

Blood substitutes:
1 True

2 True
3 True
4 False (must be given as an emulsion)

5 True

Blood donors in the UK are screened for antibodies to:
1 True
2 True
3 False
4 True
5 False

Blood storage for 2 weeks at 4–6°C:
1 True
2 True
3 False (platelets decline in the first few days)
4 True
5 False (SAGM is said to preserve erythrocyte metabolism)

Blood transfusion:

1 True

2 True (60 ml CPD and 450 ml blood)

3 True
4 False (not until 3 to 6 months of age)

5 Group A is the commonest in UK

Pages 330–331
Blood products:
1 Human albumin solution (BNF) contains no live viruses
2 Platelets may be given through a 170 μ filter
3 SAGM blood has a high viscosity
4 Red cells may be stored for years in liquid nitrogen
5 SAGM can be stored longer than CPD-A blood

Pages 332–335
Complications of blood transfusion:
1 Malaria is the commonest disease throughout the world to be transmitted by blood transfusion
2 A blood transfusion set should include a 20–40 μ filter
3 ABO incompatibility transfusion reaction is usually due to a clerical error
4 Urticaria is less common with SAGM blood
5 The temperature of a blood warming water bath may need to exceed 45°C if the transfusion is very rapid

Page 331
The following may influence crossmatching of blood:
1 Haemaccel
2 Normal saline
3 Dextran 70
4 Propofol
5 Methyldopa

Page 332
Complications of blood transfusion include:
1 Acute haemolytic reaction
2 Transmission of malaria
3 Acute heart failure
4 Immunosuppression
5 Hypernatraemia

5 False (47% O, 42% A, 8% B, 3% AB)

Blood products:
1 True
2 True (with only 5% loss. This is the common filter in giving sets)
3 False (low viscosity as it lacks plasma proteins)
4 True
5 False

Complications of blood transfusion:

1 True
2 False (of unproven value in most circumstances)

3 True
4 True (no plasma proteins)

5 False (maximum 40°C)

The following may influence crossmatching of blood:
1 False
2 False
3 True (blood bank should be informed)
4 False
5 True (blood bank should be informed)

Complications of blood transfusion include:
1 True (a grave emergency, treated like anaphylaxis)
2 True
3 True (fluid overload is a common problem)
4 True
5 False (produces hyperkalaemia; donor blood K^+ is up to 25 mmol/l)

18 Monitoring

Page 344
Damping during intra-arterial pressure monitoring:
1 Does not alter the mean arterial pressure
2 Is caused by short narrow tubing
3 Is caused by rigid tubing
4 Can be calculated by the Laplace formula
5 Is greater when the cannula is in the radial artery than in the dorsalis pedis

Pages 344–345
Pulmonary arterial catheterisation:
1 Is needed to measure SvO_2 directly
2 Was first described in man by Swan and Ganz, 1970
3 PA wedge pressure normally exceeds the CVP
4 The injectate used for measuring cardiac output by thermal dilution must be at $0°C$
5 PA wedge pressure is most reliable as an index of LA pressure if measured in the lower part of the lungs

Pages 348–349
Gas analysis:
1 N_2O influences the paramagnetic measurement of O_2
2 N_2O influences the measurement of CO_2 by a mass spectrometer
3 N_2O influences the measurement of CO_2 by an infrared analyser
4 Infrared analysis may be used to measure all the volatile agents
5 All analysers used in theatre are influenced by P_B

Page 350
Blood gases:
1 The PO_2 of blood kept in a gas-tight syringe will slowly fall
2 Gases diffuse slower through plastic than glass
3 A venous blood sample is useless for consideration of acid-base status
4 Standard HCO_3 is measured by a blood gas analyser
5 The PaO_2 of a hypothermic patient is overestimated by analysis in a machine kept at $37°C$

Damping during intra-arterial pressure monitoring:
1 True (but lowers the systolic figure)
2 False (this prevents damping)
3 False
4 False (this relates pressure to radius and surface tension)

5 False (radial and dorsalis pressures are very similar)

Pulmonary arterial catheterisation:
1 True
2 True
3 True

4 False (but a colder injectate gives a larger signal)

5 True (zone 3, where there should be a continuous column of
          blood from catheter tip to LA)

Gas analysis:
1 False
2 True (they have the same MW of 44)
3 True (but readily corrected)
4 True
5 True (they measure partial pressure, and usually have to assume
          P_B to display concentration)

Blood gases:
1 True (at about 0.4 kPa/min unless kept cold)
2 False (diffuse faster through most plastics)

3 False (it can give a useful approximation)
4 False (it is calculated)

5 True (a correction for body temperature must be made)

20 Medical diseases influencing anaesthesia

If arterial blood gases show pH 7.49; PCO_2 7.6 kPa; standard bicarbonate 34 mmol/l; base excess + 10; this could indicate:
1 Emphysema
2 An asthmatic patient getting worse
3 That 350 mmol of sodium bicarbonate has been given
4 Pyloric stenosis
5 Chronic renal failure

Wheeze:
1 Is louder during inspiration than expiration
2 Loudness is directly related to the size of the airways
3 Is more high-pitched in the larger airways
4 Is reduced by famcicylovir
5 Is relieved by H2 antagonists

Pages 374–375
Changes occurring in old age include:
1 Reduction in blood urea
2 Reduction in volume of body water
3 Reduction in arterial PO_2
4 Reduction in MAC of inhalational anaesthetics
5 Reduction in pulse pressure

Pages 375–376
Pregnancy:
1 Ranitidine is not teratogenic in humans
2 Benzodiazepines given in early pregnancy increase the incidence of cleft lip/palate
3 Aorto-caval compression is only a problem during the third trimester
4 The fetal heart may be monitored from 20 weeks
5 The lower oesophageal sphincter regains its normal competence by the second day post-partum

Page 377
The highest scoring (and risk) features in the Goldman index of cardiac risk during general surgery are:
1 Gallop rhythm

2 Aortic stenosis
3 Myocardial infarction within last 6 months
4 Age over 70 years
5 Five or more ventricular ectopics per minute

If arterial blood gases show pH 7.49; PCO$_2$ 7.6 kPa; standard bicarbonate 34 mmol/l; base excess + 10; this could indicate:
1 True
2 False (CO$_2$ usually normal or low here)
3 True (metabolic alkalosis)
4 False (does not usually produce hypercapnia)
5 False (renal failure causes acidaemia)

Wheeze:
1 False (louder in expiration)
2 False (inversely related)
3 False
4 False (this is an anti-herpes drug)
5 False (little effect on the lungs)

Changes occurring in old age include:
1 False (rises slightly)
2 True (gives a higher concentration of injected drugs)
3 True (more oxygen required during and after anaesthesia)
4 True (about 20% less at 70 years of age)
5 False (increases, mainly as systolic pressure rises)

Pregnancy:
1 True (and is useful as antacid prophylaxis)

2 True

3 False (from about 16 weeks onwards)
4 True

5 True (reduced competence from end of first trimester to second day postpartum)

The highest scoring (and risk) features in the Goldman index of cardiac risk during general surgery are:
1 True (11 points; note that > 26 points indicated a perioperative mortality of > 50%)
2 False (it is a risk, but it does not score highly in Goldman)
3 True (10 points)
4 False
5 True (7 points)

Pages 377–381
Cardiovascular disease:
1 Patients with coronary artery disease may have a normal resting ECG
2 Elective non-cardiac surgery within 3 months of a myocardial infarct is little riskier than if delayed until 6 months after the infarct

3 VT may respond to pressure on the eyeballs
4 SVT may respond to i.v. adenosine
5 HOCM is improved by beta-blockade

Page 378
A patient has a history of vomiting, epigastric pain, guarding, slight cyanosis, and surgical emphysema in the neck. Likely causes are:
1 Rupture of diaphragm
2 Spontaneous pneumothorax
3 Tear of oesophagus
4 Tear of trachea
5 Stab wound

Page 385
Asthma:
1 Inhaled steroids do not suppress adrenal function

2 Beta blockers should be avoided

3 Is often precipitated by exercise
4 Lung volumes increase during an acute episode
5 Is helped by breathing a helium-oxygen mixture

Pages 386–388
Sickle cell disease:
1 Sickling of red cells cannot occur in sickle trait
2 In sickle trait, one-third of the Hb may be HbS
3 HbS differs from HbA by a single amino acid in the beta chain
4 A Sickledex screening test for HbS is useful in patients over about 6 months of age
5 In sickle cell disease, preoperative partial exchange transfusion may be needed to reduce HbS to < 30%

Cardiovascular disease:

1 True (15% of such patients in one series)

2 False (<3 m after infarct = 25–50% re-infarction,
        3–6 m after infarct = 10–25% re-infarction,
        >6 m after infarct = about 5% re-infarction)
3 False (SVT may respond)
4 True (50–250 μg/kg, via CVP line, effect is transient)
5 True (catecholamines may make it worse)

A patient has a history of vomiting, epigastric pain, guarding, slight cyanosis, and surgical emphysema in the neck. Likely causes are:
1 False (surgical emphysema unlikely)
2 True
3 True
4 False (not likely to cause vomiting)
5 True

Asthma:
1 False (may do so with >1.5 mg beclomethasone or 6 puffs per day)
2 True (although metoprolol and atenolol are 'selective' beta blockers)
3 True (especially if the air is cold)
4 True (pneumothorax may occur rarely)
5 False (only useful if gas flow is turbulent, e.g. in upper airways obstruction)

Sickle cell disease:
1 False (may sickle if PaO_2 < about 2.7 kPa)
2 True
3 True (valine, not glutamic acid, at position 6)

4 False (over about 2 years of age)

5 True

Pages 386–388
Haemoglobinopathies:
1 Thalassaemia is common in Africans

2 Thalassaemia results in a reduced production of a particular globin chain
3 Methaemoglobin has its iron in the ferrous form
4 Methaemoglobin has a low P_{50}
5 Methylene blue is a useful reducing agent to treat methaemoglobinaemia

Pages 389–390
Treatment options in haemophilia A include:
1 Cryoprecipitate
2 Fresh frozen plasma
3 Factor VIII concentrate infused 24 hr prior to surgery
4 Tranexamic acid
5 DDAVP

Pages 391–393
Liver disease:
1 The portal vein supplies half the liver's O_2 needs
2 Hepatic artery blood flow tends to be reduced by epidural analgesia
3 Hepatic encephalopathy may be precipitated by gastric bleeding
4 The upper surface of the liver is level with the 12th thoracic vertebra
5 Plasma cholinesterase is synthesised in the liver

Pages 393–394
In the porphyrias:
1 They are commoner in South Africa than in the UK
2 The haem breakdown pathways are abnormal
3 There are abnormally high levels of ALA synthase

4 The acute intermittent form is commonest in the UK
5 Propofol has often been used safely

Pages 397–401
Diabetes mellitus:
1 An autonomic neuropathy may result
2 Hypoalbuminaemia may occur
3 A method of preoperative control is to infuse 500 ml 10% glucose with 10 units insulin and 1 g KCl at 100 ml/h

Haemoglobinopathies:
1 False (only in parts of West Africa. Typically in Mediterrancan, Middle East and S Asia)

2 True (usually the beta-chain)
3 False (ferric; ferrous is normal)
4 True (less able to give O_2 to the tissues)

5 True (dose is 1–2 mg/kg of 1% solution)

Treatment options in haemophilia A include:
1 True
2 True
3 False (biological half-life < 12 hr)
4 True (inhibits fibrinolysis)
5 True (synthetic vasopressin)

Liver disease:
1 True

2 True (but also by general anaesthesia)
3 True (protein load increases blood ammonia)

4 False (usually level with T10)
5 True

In the porphyrias:
1 True
2 False (inborn errors of haem synthesis)
3 True (the rate-limiting enzyme in the synthesis of haem and is normally inhibited by it)
4 True
5 True

Diabetes mellitus:
1 True (giving unstable cardiovascular system)
2 True (the nephropathy may cause nephrotic syndrome)

3 True (an 'Alberti' regime)

4 The action of tolbutamide lasts more than 24 hr
5 Hypoglycaemia may be induced by beta-blockers

Pages 404–405
Carcinoid syndrome:
1 Only occurs if there are liver metastases
2 Typical features are headache and a labile BP
3 Confirmed by a 24 hr urinary HIAA of > 25 mg
4 May result in tricuspid and pulmonary stenoses
5 Octreotide is a useful treatment

Page 405
Steroid hormones:
1 Secretion of hydrocortisone is normally 20 mg/day
2 Secretion of hydrocortisone may rise to 500 mg/day with extreme stress
3 Steroid cover is not needed after a course of steroid therapy for less than 2 weeks
4 Steroid cover should be given even if steroid therapy ended 2 weeks previously
5 Dexamethasone is 30 times as potent a glucocorticoid as hydrocortisone

Pages 406–408
Difficult intubation may be a feature of the following connective tissue disorders:
1 Rheumatoid arthritis
2 Ankylosing spondylitis
3 Polyarteritis nodosa
4 SLE
5 Achondroplasia

Restrictive lung function tests may occur in:
1 Rheumatoid arthritis
2 Ankylosing spondylitis
3 Polyarteritis nodosa
4 SLE
5 Achondroplasia

Pages 408–411
Myasthenia gravis:
1 Is associated with muscle pains

4 False (8 hr; chlorpropamide exceeds 24 hr)
5 True

Carcinoid syndrome:
1 True (they can be very slow-growing)
2 False (flushing, wheezing and diarrhoea)
3 True
4 True (may need heart surgery)
5 True (analogue of somatostatin which suppresses secretion of 5HT)

Steroid hormones:
1 True

2 True

3 False (adrenal suppression may occur after just 1 week)

4 True (adrenal suppression is likely to occur up to 2 months after the end of therapy)

5 True

Difficult intubation may be a feature of the following connective tissue disorders:
1 True (cervical spine and T-M joint immobility)
2 True (cervical spine and T-M joint immobility)
3 False (but renal, cardiac, pulmonary involvement)
4 False
5 True (limited head extension)

Restrictive lung function tests may occur in:
1 True (due to rib-cage stiffness)
2 True (due to rib-cage stiffness)
3 True (due to pulmonary involvement)
4 True (due to pleural effusion)
5 True (due to rib abnormalities)

Myasthenia gravis:
1 False (more typical of myasthenic syndrome)

2 Can present at any age
3 Is commoner in men
4 Symptoms often worsen for up to 4 months after childbirth
5 Is often worsened by aminoglycoside antibiotics

The following features distinguish myasthenic (Eaton–Lambert) syndrome (ELS) from myasthenia gravis (MG):
1 Diminished tendon reflexes
2 Commonly affects extra-ocular muscles

3 Relative resistance to suxamethonium

4 Abnormal motor nerve terminals

5 A poor prognosis

Pages 411–414
Diseases of the nervous system:
1 Propofol has been used to treat status epilepticus
2 Relapses of multiple sclerosis are commoner following childbirth
3 Motor neurone disease causes cardiomyopathy
4 Cardiomyopathy is a feature of Duchenne muscular dystrophy
5 Malignant hyperpyrexia is more common in patients with muscular dystrophy

Dystrophia myotonica:
1 Is inherited as an autosomal recessive
2 The myotonia is relieved by relaxants

3 Muscle fibre membranes are abnormal
4 Cardiomyopathy is commonly associated
5 Extradural block is contraindicated

Page 391
Hepatic encephalopathy in cirrhotics is caused by:
1 Barbiturates
2 Constipation
3 Oral neomycin
4 Surgery
5 Bleeding varices

2 True (usually in early adulthood)
3 False (twice as common in women)
4 True
5 True

The following features distinguish myasthenic (Eaton–Lambert) syndrome (ELS) from myasthenia gravis (MG):
1 True
2 False (MG affects these and the bulbar muscles; while ELS affects proximal limb muscles)
3 False (true for MG, but ELS shows increased sensitivity to all relaxants)
4 True (IgG antibodies to voltage-gated Ca^{++} channels in the terminals with reduced release of ACh)
5 True (associated with small cell Ca bronchus)

Diseases of the nervous system:
1 True (with successful results)
2 True (pyrexias also cause relapses)
3 False (it is not caused by motor neurone disease)
4 True (cardiac arrest may occur during anaesthesia)

5 True

Dystrophia myotonica:
1 False (autosomal dominant)
2 False (precipitated by depolarisers, unaffected by non-depolarisers)
3 True (abnormal Cl^- conductance)
4 True
5 False (has been used with success)

Hepatic encephalopathy in cirrhotics is caused by:
1 False
2 True (by promoting fermentation in the gut)
3 False (prevents fermentation in the gut)
4 True (by causing protein catabolism)
5 True (by giving large protein load in gut)

22 Surgical operations and choice of anaesthetic

Cardio-thoracic surgery

Pages 451–461
In open-chest surgery:
1 An open pneumothorax causes pendelluft if the patient is breathing spontaneously
2 Such pendelluft is worsened by IPPV
3 The right upper lobe bronchus orifice is much closer to the carina than the left upper lobe bronchus
4 Suction applied postoperatively to a pleural drain should not exceed about 5 cm H_2O
5 An empyema is best drained under LA

During pulmonary surgery:
1 Nitrous oxide is a useful agent with large lung bullae
2 Anaphylaxis is common if a hydatid cyst ruptures
3 Transplanted lungs tend to become oedematous
4 A bronchopleural fistula (BPF) may make IPPV through a tracheal tube ineffective
5 BPF can result in infected secretions flooding the 'good' lung

The hypoxaemia of one-lung anaesthesia may be improved by:
1 Increasing tidal volume
2 PEEP
3 Insufflation of O_2 in the upper lung
4 CPAP to the upper lung
5 Clamping the pulmonary artery to the lower lung

Bronchoscopy:
1 A bronchial foreign body is best removed with a fibreoptic bronchoscope
2 Can be done under deep inhalational anaesthesia
3 When recovering from a bronchial biopsy, a patient should be placed with the side of the biopsy lowermost
4 Rigid bronchoscopy has lesser haemodynamic effects than intubation using a Macintosh laryngoscope
5 Trans-cricoid injection of local anaesthetic is necessary for fibreoptic bronchoscopy in an awake patient

In open-chest surgery:

1 True
2 False (pendelluft is prevented by IPPV)

3 True

4 True
5 True

During pulmonary surgery:
1 False (it will enlarge them further)
2 True (hypotension and bronchospasm are seen)
3 True (their lymphatics have been severed)

4 True (although the air leak is usually small)
5 True

The hypoxaemia of one-lung anaesthesia may be improved by:
1 True (but if too high, blood flow is diverted to the upper, unventilated lung)
2 True (but worsened if blood flow is diverted)
3 True
4 True (but this may impede surgical access)
5 False (by clamping the pulmonary artery to the upper lung)

Bronchoscopy:

1 False (a rigid bronchoscope is preferred)
2 True (especially in children)

3 True (to prevent soiling the other lung)

4 False (more, and for a longer time)

5 False (but used by some practitioners; local analgesic can also be injected via the bronchoscope)

Pages 462–464

Closed cardiac surgery:

1 Cardiopulmonary bypass is needed to ligate a patent ductus arteriosus
2 Clamping the aorta for coarctation surgery in an adult gives less rise in blood pressure than in a child
3 Aortic coarctation is associated with berry aneurysms in the cerebral circulation
4 Ischaemia of the spinal cord is a risk of surgery for coarctation
5 Pulsus alternans may be caused by pericarditis

Open cardiac surgery

Pages 464–469

During cardiopulmonary bypass:

1 The arterial pressure is usually adjusted by altering the speed of the roller pump
2 The desired flow through the aortic cannula is usually calculated before surgery
3 The heart consumes more O_2 during ventricular fibrillation (VF) than during asystole
4 On cooling, VF occurs at about 32°C
5 The haematocrit is kept normal

Anticoagulation (and its reversal) during cardiopulmonary bypass:

1 Is achieved with acid citrate dextrose
2 Is measured by the activated clotting time (ACT)
3 The 'activated' in ACT refers to the celite accelerator
4 Protamine allergy is related to fish allergy
5 Protamine can cause severe hypertension

Complications of cardiopulmonary bypass include:

1 Phrenic nerve palsy
2 Bubble emboli
3 Postoperative hyperthermia
4 Haemolysis
5 Awareness

Closed cardiac surgery:

1 False (usually performed through a left thoracotomy)

2 True (better developed collaterals)

3 True
4 True (especially in children)
5 False (pericarditis may cause *pulsus paradoxus*)

During cardiopulmonary bypass:

1 False (by giving vaso-constrictors or dilators)

2 True (about 2 l/sq.m/min)

3 True
4 False (nearer 28°C)
5 False (lowered to 20–25% by the 'priming' solution
    in the bypass circuit)

Anticoagulation (and its reversal) during cardiopulmonary bypass:
1 False (heparin 300 units/kg)
2 True
3 True
4 True (protamine is a fish-roe product)
5 False (hypotension is common; protamine should be
    injected slowly)

Complications of cardiopulmonary bypass include:
1 True (from cold solutions applied to the heart)
2 True (bypasses have traps to prevent this)
3 False (hypothermia, from uneven re-warming)
4 True (due to erythrocyte damage in roller pumps)
5 True (especially on discontinuing bypass)

Surgery of the endocrine glands

Pages 487–492
In surgery of the thyroid gland:
1   Lugol's iodine reduces vascularity of the gland
2   Carbimazole reduces vascularity of the gland
3   The recurrent laryngeal nerve is usually seen
4   The superior laryngeal nerve is never damaged
5   Beta-blockers are useful in the thyrotoxic patient

Phaeochromocytoma:
1   Is often not diagnosed
2   Is localised with the help of an abdominal CT scan
3   Localisation is secure if a mass is seen in one adrenal medulla
4   Meta-iodobenzylguanidine scanning is useful
5   After excision, hyperglycaemia often results

Phaeochromocytoma:
1   May be part of multiple endocrine neoplasia type I
2   Occur outside the adrenal medulla in 10% of cases
3   Is not a malignant tumour
4   May cause a cardiomyopathy
5   During preparation for surgery, beta-blockade should be started before alpha-blockade

Neurosurgery

Pages 492–507
In operations on the brain:
1   A short period of straining may cause cerebral oedema lasting for hours
2   The endotracheal tube should be secured with tapes
3   PEEP is undesirable
4   The brain may be exposed under local analgesia
5   Conventional laryngoscopy may increase cerebral venous pressure

The normal adult brain:
1   Occupies 95% of the cranium
2   Weighs 750 g
3   Has a blood flow of about 1.5 l/min
4   Grey matter is more vascular than white matter

In surgery of the thyroid gland:
1 True (dose 0.3 ml three times daily)
2 False (it increases vascularity)
3 True (but the nerve may have several branches)
4 False (this injury is well recognised)
5 True (to prevent arrhythmias and calm the patient)

Phaeochromocytoma:
1 True (due to the intermittent nature of the symptoms)
2 True (more than one tumour may be present)
3 False (10% are bilateral)
4 True
5 False (the blood sugar may well fall, especially if the patient is
       on beta-blockers)

Phaeochromocytoma:
1 False (types II and III)
2 True
3 False (about 10% of these are malignant)
4 True

5 False (this can *increase* the blood pressure)

In operations on the brain:

1 True
2 False (tapes may obstruct the neck veins)
3 True (raises cerebral venous pressure)
4 True

5 True

The normal adult brain:
1 False (80% brain, 12% blood, 8% CSF)
2 False (1500 g)
3 False (750 ml/min, or 15% of cardiac output)
4 True (70 and 20 ml/min/100 g respectively)

5 Oxygen consumption is about 50 ml/min

Blood flow to the normal brain:
1 Doubles if the normal $PaCO_2$ is doubled
2 Is nearly constant as the cerebral perfusion pressure increases from about 50 to 150 mmHg
3 Is extremely sensitive to autonomic nervous activity
4 Increases in fever
5 If less than 40% of normal causes EEG changes

Anaesthetic agents in neurosurgery:
1 Intravenous induction agents reduce cerebral blood flow
2 Narcotic analgesics increase cerebral blood flow
3 Nitrous oxide decreases cerebral blood flow
4 Of the volatile agents, halothane is the most potent cerebral vasodilator

5 Isoflurane can produce a flat EEG at 2 MAC

Raised intracranial pressure (ICP):
1 May be progressively reduced by hyperventilation down to a PCO_2 of 2 kPa (15 mmHg)

2 Is lowered only for a limited time by hyperventilation

3 Is reduced by head-up tilt
4 If due to tumour, dexamethasone is of value
5 Is reduced within minutes by i.v. mannitol

Complications of surgery in the posterior cranial fossa include:
1 Hydrocephalus
2 Asystole
3 Swelling of the tongue
4 Anosmia
5 Bulbar palsy

Air embolism during surgery on a patient in the sitting position:
1 Cannot occur before the skull is opened

2 If resuscitation is needed the patient should be placed on his left side
3 May be detected by a sudden fall in end-tidal CO_2
4 Is worsened by the administration of nitrous oxide

5 True (about 20% of the whole body's consumption)

Blood flow to the normal brain:
1 True (this makes $PaCO_2$ control very important)

2 True (autoregulation)
3 False
4 True (about 10% increase per extra °C)
5 True

Anaesthetic agents in neurosurgery:
1 True (except ketamine, which increases it)
2 False (they have little effect)
3 False (probably tends to increase it slightly)

4 True (cerebral blood flow tripled at 1 MAC, but only doubled with this concentration of enflurane and no change with isoflurane)
5 True

Raised intracranial pressure (ICP):

1 False (vasoconstriction in the brain is nearly maximal at 3.5 kPa, or 26 mmHg)
2 True (the ICP increases again over 24 hr despite the hyperventilation)
3 True
4 True
5 True (but this effect wears off in a few hours)

Complications of surgery in the posterior cranial fossa include:
1 True (obstruction of the 4th ventricle)
2 True
3 True
4 False (the olfactory nerve is at the front of the brain)
5 True

Air embolism during surgery on a patient in the sitting position:
1 False (air may enter through the venous plexus in the occipital muscles)

2 True (directs air away from the pulmonary artery)
3 True (it prevents pulmonary excretion of CO_2)
4 True (it diffuses into the bubbles and enlarges them)

5   Is unlikely to be paradoxical

Page 505
The magnetic field used for magnetic resonance imaging can:
1   Attract laryngoscope batteries
2   Induce small electric currents in blood vessels
3   Cause T-wave changes in the ECG
4   Cause electronic circuits to malfunction
5   Cause erythema and itching in some skin tattoos

Page 506
In electro-convulsive therapy (ECT):
1   Propofol shortens the 'fit' of ECT
2   Causes mild and transient cardiovascular changes
3   Causes no visible change if the patient is completely paralysed
4   Can be given in mid-pregnancy with safety
5   Provided the first clinical use of muscle relaxants

Pages 507–510
In head injury:
1   The extent of brain injury may be increased if there is hyperglycaemia
2   The Glasgow coma score is calculated from observation of best verbal and motor responses
3   A Glasgow coma score of 1 is better than one of 14
4   Fits are of little consequence in a paralysed patient
5   No established measures protect the brain against the consequences of ischaemic injury after it has occurred

In 'brainstem death':
1   There is a 'doll's-eye reflex'
2   A basic diagnosis must be established
3   An EEG should be performed for confirmation
4   Two examinations of the patient are needed, at least 24 hours apart
5   The 'time of death' is the end of the second test

In the management of a patient who is brainstem dead, and is acting as an organ donor:
1   Diabetes insipidus may have to be treated
2   Movement in response to incision indicates that the diagnosis of brainstem death was incorrect
3   Monitoring during surgery is not needed
4   Cardiac output should be optimised

5 False (air often traverses a patent foramen ovale)

The magnetic field used for magnetic resonance imaging can:
1 True
2 True (of no consequence)
3 True (of no clinical significance)
4 True
5 True (if metallic dyes have been used)

In electro-convulsive therapy (ECT):
1 True (but does it reduce its clinical efficacy?)
2 True (it is almost impossible to monitor these)
3 False (pilomotor reaction, absent pupillary light reflex)
4 True
5 True (curare in 1940)

In head injury:

1 True

2 False (also includes observation of eye opening)
3 False (the low numbers are the worse responses)
4 False (they greatly increase brain O_2 consumption)

5 True

In 'brainstem death':
1 False (not compatible with brainstem death)
2 True
3 False

4 False (the interval should be 'clinically appropriate')
5 True

In the management of a patient who is brainstem dead, and is acting as an organ donor:
1 True (with a vasopressin analogue, e.g. DDAVP)

2 False (spinal reflexes may occur)
3 False
4 True

5 Dopamine infusion may be needed

In spinal injury:
1 Respiratory reserve is best assessed by vital capacity
2 Section of the cord at C3 will mean total dependence
   on artificial ventilation at all times

3 Some weeks after the injury, autonomic hyperreflexia may
   occur in response to painful stimuli
4 Spinal anaesthesia prevents autonomic hyperreflexia
5 Suxamethonium is safe one month after the injury

Obstetrics

Pages 512–537
Fetal suxamethonium levels are low because:
1 A low dose is usually injected into the mother
2 Suxamethonium has an elongated molecule
3 The fetus is surrounded by liquor amnii
4 The placenta contains large amounts of cholinesterase
5 Suxamethonium is highly ionised

Pages 533–535
**Causes of a floppy baby during anaesthesia for Caesarean
section are:**
1 Use of suxamethonium
2 Placental failure
3 Taking longer than 2 minutes from incision of uterus to delivery
4 Severe prematurity
5 Maternal hyperkalaemia

Fetal blood levels of thiopentone are:
1 Higher than in the mother
2 Around 35–70 micrograms per ml
3 Around 3.5–7 micrograms per ml
4 Maximal in the umbilical vein around 1 min after injection
5 Related to the serum potassium concentration

5 True

In spinal injury:
1 True

2 False (patients may be taught to manipulate their pharyngeal muscles and 'swallow' air into their lungs)

3 True (may even occur with a full bladder)
4 True
5 False (may result in hyperkalaemia at this time)

Fetal suxamethonium levels are low because:
1 False (normal or high doses are used)
2 False
3 False
4 False (but the placenta is rich in cholinesterase)
5 True (its quarternary amine groups reduce placental transfer)

Causes of a floppy baby during anaesthesia for Caesarean section are:
1 False (it does not cross the placenta)
2 True (often the reason for the 'section')
3 True (incision reduces placental perfusion)
4 True
5 False (no relation to floppy babies)

Fetal blood levels of thiopentone are:
1 False (they are lower than in the mother)
2 False
3 True (F/M ratio 0.45–1)
4 True
5 False

Plastic surgery

Pages 590–592
In burns:
1   According to the 'rule of nines', the trunk accounts for just over a third of the body surface area of an adult
2   If over 30% , the patient is unlikely to survive
3   If there is any evidence of respiratory burns, the airway should be secured *immediately* by intubation
4   Large amounts of intravenous colloid are needed

5   There are very large energy requirements

Urology

Pages 595–599
In transurethral resection of the prostate:
1   Water is used to irrigate the bladder during surgery
2   Several litres of irrigant may be absorbed
3   A 'saddle' spinal block provides good analgesia

4   Hypothermia may result if the irrigant is not warmed
5   Transient blindness may occur

Complications of nephrectomy include:
1   Pneumothorax
2   Hypotension when the renal artery is clamped
3   Intraoperative pulmonary embolus
4   Hypoxaemia during surgery
5   Peripheral nerve injury

In burns:

1 True (front and back are 18% each)
2 False (nearer 60%, except in the elderly)

3 True (oral oedema, carbon in sputum, hypoxaemia)
4 True (e.g. 0.5 × weight (kg) × burn area (%) in ml
given every 4 hr for the first 12 hr)
5 True (20 kcal/kg + 50 kcal/% burn, per day)

In transurethral resection of the prostate:
1 False (1.5% glycine solution is commonest in UK)
2 True (causing the TURP syndrome)
3 False (block must ascend at least to T10, to cover distension of
the bladder)
4 True (and can be severe)
5 True (glycine is an inhibitory neurotransmitter)

Complications of nephrectomy include:
1 True (tension pneumothorax in laparoscopic nephrectomy)
2 False (hypertension if there is a vascular tumour)
3 True (tumour can extend up the IVC)
4 True (lateral position)
5 True (lateral position)

23 Anaesthesia in abnormal environments

Pages 603–608
In anaesthesia given at high altitude:
1 Nitrous oxide is a valuable adjunct to anaesthesia administered at an altitude of 5,000 feet

2 Cylinder pressure gauges are accurate
3 Rotameters over-read at altitude
4 Vaporisers at the same dial setting deliver the same partial pressure of the vapour whatever the altitude
5 An O_2 analyser will read accurately at all altitudes

In anaesthesia given at high altitude:

1 False (too high a concentration causes hypoxia,
        and the partial pressure is less anyway)
2 True
3 False (low gas density allows the bobbin to fall)

4 True (SVP does not change with altitude)
5 False (all gas analysers used in operating theatres vary with
        partial pressure)

24 Regional analgesia

Pages 628–744
Before regional analgesia:
1 Skin cleaning is not necessary
2 A defibrillator should be available
3 Infiltration of local anaesthetic is essential

4 Premedication is essential
5 Consent is required

Page 618
Toxicity of local anaesthetics is influenced by:
1 Concentration of drug
2 Volume of solution injected
3 Presence of adrenaline

4 Site of injection
5 Carbonation of drug

Page 623
Lignocaine:
1 Is antibacterial
2 Is an ester-linked chemical
3 Is slow in onset
4 Is absorbed in mucous membranes
5 Maximum safe injection dose in tissues is 3 mg/kg

Lignocaine:
1 Stabilises the myocardium
2 Is not absorbed from the trachea
3 Overdose can be treated by diazepam
4 Is a drug of addiction
5 0.5% blocks motor fibres

Page 625
Bupivacaine:
1 Is less toxic than lignocaine
2 Has faster onset than prilocaine
3 Prevents cardiac arrhythmias
4 Block with 0.75% lasts longer than 0.125%
5 Is an amide

Before regional analgesia:
1 False (skin cleaning is essential)
2 True (full resuscitation equipment is needed)
3 False (may be rendered painless by freezing with
      snow or ice in an emergency)
4 False (desirable but not essential)
5 True

Toxicity of local anaesthetics is influenced by:
1 True (the higher the concentration, the more toxic)
2 True (the larger the volume, the more toxic)
3 True (adrenaline tends to reduce the toxicity,
      except if the injection is intravenous)
4 True (toxicity more likely in vascular sites)
5 False (no effect)

Lignocaine:
1 True (a little-known but useful effect)
2 False (an amide chemical)
3 False (the fastest in common use)
4 True (excellent for topical use)
5 True (this allows for absorption from very vascular sites; the
      figure could be doubled if adrenaline is used)

1 True (used to control ectopic beats)
2 False (rapidly absorbed)
3 True (to control convulsions)
4 False (cocaine is the addictive local anaesthetic)
5 False (1.5–2% needed for this; 0.5% blocks the smaller
      autonomic and sensory fibres)

1 False (maximum safe dose is 2 mg/kg)
2 False (much slower – may take 30 min)
3 False (causes cardiac arrhythmias when given i.v.)
4 True (much less difference between 0.25% and 0.5%)
5 True

Pages 625–626
Prilocaine:
1   Is less toxic than bupivacaine
2   Is metabolised in the kidneys
3   Is metabolised in the lungs
4   Methaemoglobinaemia makes the patient look blue

5   Methaemoglobinaemia produces hypoxia

Page 626
Ropivacaine:
1   Gives better motor block than bupivacaine
2   If given with adrenaline gives lower blood levels after tissue injection
3   Is less cardiotoxic than bupivacaine
4   Is shorter acting than prilocaine
5   Is destroyed by gamma radiation

Page 631
Maxillary nerve block:
1   Is suitable for operations on forehead

2   The needle is inserted above the zygoma
3   The needle is advanced towards the opposite eyeball
4   Aspiration of air indicates the right direction
5   Causes nasal vasodilation

Page 633
Moffett's block:
1   Is inserted with patient sitting up
2   Blocks the geniculate ganglion
3   Bupivacaine is the drug of choice

4   Produces sympathetic blockade of nose
5   Moffett's solution contains 8% $NaHCO_3$

Page 635
Mandibular nerve block:
1   Is suitable for extraction of upper 1st molar
2   Is suitable for extraction of lower central incisor
3   The needle is inserted by the internal oblique ridge
4   The syringe lies over the opposite premolar
5   The block extends from the chin to the tongue

Prilocaine:
1   True (prilocaine is one of the safest local anaesthetics)
2   True
3   True
4   True (although prilocaine rarely produces enough to make
        this happen)
5   True (shifts the O_2 dissociation curve to the left)

Ropivacaine:
1   True (using equal concentrations)

2   False (no effect, unlike other local anaesthetics)
3   True
4   False (is equal to bupivacaine)
5   False (stable in gamma radiation)

Maxillary nerve block:
1   False (for cheek, lower eyelid, nose, antrum, palate, upper teeth.
        Forehead is supplied by ophthalmic division)
2   False (below the zygoma)
3   True
4   True (it indicates needle tip has entered nose)
5   False (vasoconstriction due to parasympathetic block)

Moffett's block:
1   False (supine, and head 45° down)
2   False (blocks sphenopalatine ganglion)
3   False (cocaine 8%, which is absorbed through the nasal mucous
        membrane)
4   False (parasympathetic blockade of nose)
5   False (1% $NaHCO_3$)

Mandibular nerve block:
1   False (mandibular nerve supplies lower teeth)
2   False (lower central incisor has contralateral innervation)
3   True
4   True
5   True

Page 637
Stellate ganglion block:
1 Blocks the splanchnic nerve
2 Produces sympathetic block of the arm
3 Produces Mueller's syndrome
4 Produces Horner's syndrome

5 Prevents sweating in that side of the neck

Page 640
Cervical plexus block:
1 Gives analgesia down to elbows
2 Gives analgesia up to top of head

3 Requires needle to point slightly caudally to prevent vertebral artery puncture
4 Requires needle to point slightly caudally to prevent epidural block
5 Analgesic drug is placed in the interscalene sheath

Page 646
Interscalene approach to the brachial plexus:
1 Injection is made above the level of the cricoid
2 May also block the cervical plexus
3 Adult requires an analgesic volume of 10 ml
4 May cause pneumothorax
5 Suitable for operations on the wrist joint

Supraclavicular perivascular brachial plexus block:
1 May cause pneumothorax
2 May cause arterial injection
3 May cause venous injection
4 Is not suitable for operations on wrist
5 Shoulder paraesthesia indicates correct needle placement

Page 647
Axillary brachial plexus block:
1 Blocks musculocutaneous nerve

2 Is suitable for operations on shoulder

Stellate ganglion block:
1 False (the splanchnic nerve is in the abdomen)
2 True (except for the nerve of Kuntz)
3 True (facial warmth and tympanic redness)
4 True (ptosis, miosis, enophthalmos, hyperaemia and anhydrosis)
5 True (by blocking sympathetic nerves)

Cervical plexus block:
1 False (down to clavicles)
2 False (up to occiput; ophthalmic division of trigeminal nerve supplies top of head)

3 True (prevents needle going between transverse processes)

4 True (prevents needle going between transverse processes)
5 True

Interscalene approach to the brachial plexus:
1 False (below the cricoid)
2 True (analgesic spreads up as well as down)
3 False (30 ml)
4 False (safe if done at C6)
5 True (but large volumes of analgesic are needed)

Supraclavicular perivascular brachial plexus block:
1 True (needle tip is very close to pleura)
2 True (needle tip is very close to subclavian artery)
3 True (needle tip is very close to subclavian vein)
4 False (it produces widespread block)
5 False (this is due to suprascapular nerve irritation)

Axillary brachial plexus block:
1 False (this leaves the sheath high in the axilla and may be missed)
2 False (the intercostohumeral and suprascapular nerves are not blocked)

3 Is suitable for operations on wrist
4 The needle is inserted posterior to biceps
5 Is suitable for arm tourniquets

Page 649

Intravenous regional analgesia (IVRA):
1 Can be used in the leg
2 Requires 2 intravenous cannulae
3 Cuff is inflated just above the mean blood pressure
4 Bupivacaine is the best analgesic for IVRA
5 Used in patients with sickle cell disease

Page 652

Wrist block:
1 Involves musculocutaneous nerve
2 Indicated in carpal tunnel syndrome
3 Not suitable for operations on palm
4 Radial nerve is blocked on shaft of radius
5 Ulnar nerve is blocked at wrist crease

Page 654

Lumbar sympathetic block:
1 Needles are inserted over spinous processes
2 If needle tip strikes transverse process, it is angled laterally
3 Aortic injection is a risk
4 Inferior vena cava is safe from injection
5 Indicated in arterial insufficiency of feet

Page 663

Abdominal field block:
1 Is simply an intramuscular block
2 Paralyses the abdominal wall
3 Analgesia of the abdominal wall is complete
4 Causes coughing
5 May cause pneumothorax

Page 666

Ilio-inguinal nerve block:
1 Blocks nerves from roots L2–5
2 Volume of analgesic needed in an adult is 5 ml

3 True
4 True
5 False (this may need subcutaneous injection of lignocaine to make it comfortable)

Intravenous regional analgesia (IVRA):
1 True (but needs larger doses)
2 True (one on contralateral side for emergencies)
3 False (well above systolic pressure)
4 False (most cardiotoxic and not used)
5 False (the limb hypoxia causes local sickling)

Wrist block:
1 False (median, ulnar and radial nerves)
2 False (unwise in cases of neuritis)
3 False (produces good block of palm)
4 True (2 cm above radial styloid)
5 False (it divides above this and should be blocked proximal to crease)

Lumbar sympathetic block:
1 False (5–10 cm lateral to spinous processes)
2 False (it is angled upwards and medially)
3 True (if needle goes too far in on the left)
4 False (equally at risk on the right side)
5 True (it sometimes improves rest pain)

Abdominal field block:
1 False (subcutaneous branches need blocking as well)
2 True (very useful in laparotomies)
3 True
4 False (it weakens coughing)
5 True (but only if needle strays above costal margin)

Ilio-inguinal nerve block:
1 False (T12 and L1)
2 False (20 ml or more usually required)

3 Ilio-inguinal nerve lies lateral to anterior superior iliac spine
4 Block of ilio-inguinal, ilio-hypogastric and genito-femoral nerves is all that is needed for herniorrhaphy
5 Unsuitable for post-operative analgesia

Page 670
Penile block:
1 Makes the penis smaller
2 Adrenaline must not be used
3 Dorsal nerves are blocked in the corpus cavernosum
4 Bupivacaine must not be used
5 Ventral nerves of penis should be blocked when using penile block for circumcision

Page 677
Psoas compartment block:
1 Is approached from the groin
2 Uses the upper border of L4 as a landmark
3 Adult requires 10 ml of analgesic solution
4 Gives analgesia of the hip joint
5 Can produce bilateral block

Page 678
Ankle block:
1 Peroneal nerve is blocked in front of ankle joint
2 Sural nerve is blocked between lateral malleolus and the Achilles tendon
3 Saphenous nerve is blocked at neck of fibula

4 Tibial nerve is blocked posterior to lateral malleolus
5 Is suitable for Potts' fracture

A lumbar vertebra has:
1 A body anteriorly
2 A laminar arch posteriorly
3 Discs superiorly and inferiorly
4 Muscles all round it
5 Facetal joints on the laminae

Page 693
The spinal canal:
1 Is widest in the thoracic region
2 Is bounded anteriorly by the anterior longitudinal ligament
3 Dura stops at L1/2

3 False (1 fingerbreadth medial to it)

4 False (hernial sac also needs infiltrating for herniorrhaphy)
5 False (it is very suitable)

Penile block:
1 False (often larger, but flaccid)
2 True (risk of gangrene)
3 False (between corpus cavernosum and symphysis)
4 False (its long action is desirable)

5 True (these are branches of pudendal nerves)

Psoas compartment block:
1 False (groin approach is for 3 in 1 block)
2 True (level with posterior iliac spine)
3 False (usually 40 ml)
4 True
5 True

Ankle block:
1 True (below the tibia, above the talus)

2 True
3 False (blocked in front of medial malleolus, close to saphenous vein)
4 False (posterior to medial malleolus)
5 False (suitable for operations below ankle joint)

A lumbar vertebra has:
1 True
2 True
3 True
4 False (aorta and IVC are anterior relations)
5 True

The spinal canal:
1 False (lumbar)
2 False (posterior longitudinal ligament)
3 False (cord stops at L1/2)

4 Dura stops at S1/2
5 Veins in the spinal canal drain into azygos system

Page 700
Complications of thoraco-lumbar epidural blockade include:
1 Hypertension
2 Headache
3 Backache
4 Vertebral osteoporosis
5 Tachycardia

Before starting an epidural block:
1 Blood glucose level is needed
2 A defibrillator should be nearby
3 Intravenous cannulation is not necessary
4 The skin must be cleaned
5 X-ray of spine must be seen

Pages 701 and 712
The following are helpful in management of hypotension in epidural block:
1 Head-up tilt
2 Thiopentone
3 CO_2
4 Metoclopromide
5 Ephedrine

Page 713
Spinal needles:
1 The Sprotte needle has a side orifice
2 The Whitacre needle has an end orifice
3 The Tuohy needle has a Huber point

4 The Labat needle has a long bevel
5 The Lee needle has centimetre markings on it

Page 717
Central neural blockade is avoided in a patient:
1 For a massive ovarian cystectomy
2 For a colectomy
3 With aortic stenosis

4 With intracranial hypotension

4 True
5 True

Complications of thoraco-lumbar epidural blockade include:
1 False (hypotension due to sympathetic blockade)
2 True (even in the absence of dural puncture)
3 True (especially in labour when motor block has been produced)
4 False
5 False (block of sympathetic drive to the heart)

Before starting an epidural block:
1 False (blood glucose is well maintained)
2 True (full resuscitation equipment available)
3 False (this is essential, see Synopsis, page 711)
4 True (don't forget to mention this in exams!)
5 False (can be helpful, but not essential)

The following are helpful in management of hypotension in epidural block:
1 False (head down tilt encourages venous return)
2 False (lowers arterial pressure even further)
3 False (but oxygen is very important)
4 True (hypotension is often associated with nausea)
5 True (alpha and beta agonist effects make this a very useful drug)

Spinal needles:
1 True
2 False (side; pencil point needle)
3 True (a rounded point intended to part the fibres of ligaments, but not to pierce the dura)
4 False (short bevel)
5 True (the original marked needle)

Central neural blockade is avoided in a patient:
1 True (because of severe hypotension)
2 False (provides good operating conditions)
3 True (unable to cope with vasodilation because of fixed cardiac output)
4 False (avoided in intracranial hypertension)

5 With Plummer–Vinson syndrome

Page 717
Epidural block is unwise in:
1 Perforated peptic ulcer
2 Bedsores
3 Dehydrated patients
4 Patients in whom the INR is 1.3

5 Disseminated intravascular coagulopathy

Page 735
Spinal opioids:
1 Relieve ischaemic pain
2 Morphine spreads further than fentanyl
3 Can be given safely with parenteral opioids
4 Act on mu receptors in posterior horn
5 Cause itching

5 False (it may prevent regurgitation; Synopsis, page 435)

Epidural block is unwise in:
1 True (vasodilation causes severe hypotension in shock)
2 True (risk of spinal infection)
3 True (vasodilation causes severe hypotension)
4 False (probably no increased risk of haematoma if the INR is under 2)
5 True (epidural haematoma is a risk)

Spinal opioids:
1 True
2 True (the more water soluble morphine diffuses in the CSF)
3 False (increased risk of apnoea)
4 False (kappa receptors)
5 True

26 Acute pain

Page 750
Postoperative pain:
1 Is worst in thoracic operations
2 Is worse in the evening
3 Causes atelectasis
4 Is improved by movement
5 Causes acidosis

Page 751
Non-steroidal anti-inflammatory drugs (NSAIDs):
1 Increase synthesis of prostaglandin E
2 May worsen renal failure
3 Reduce stickiness of platelets
4 May cause penile ulceration
5 May cause fluid retention

Page 759
Pethidine:
1 Causes more biliary colic than fentanyl
2 Is more lipophilic than fentanyl
3 Has a faster onset than fentanyl
4 Causes more vasodilation than fentanyl
5 Causes more bronchospasm than fentanyl

Page 762
Naloxone:
1 Has mu receptor affinity
2 Has mu receptor efficacy
3 Lowers the arterial pressure in septic shock
4 Reverses the analgesia of intrathecal morphine
5 Improves performance in alcohol intoxication

Postoperative pain:
1 True
2 True
3 True (because of shallow respiration and impaired coughing)
4 False (worsened by movement)
5 False (most often a respiratory alkalosis)

Non-steroidal anti-inflammatory drugs (NSAIDs):
1 False (inhibit synthesis of PGE)
2 True
3 True
4 False (cause peptic ulceration)
5 True

Pethidine:
1 False (pethidine does not cause colic)
2 False (less lipophilic)
3 True (especially after i.m. injection)
4 True
5 False (pethidine is a bronchodilator)

Naloxone:
1 True
2 False (this is why it is an opioid antagonist)
3 False (raises it, suggesting endorphin involvement)
4 False
5 True (very useful!)

27 Non-acute pain

Page 766
The following factors modify non-acute pain:
1 Acid-base status
2 Depression
3 Hope
4 Sex of patient
5 Time of day

Page 769
The following drugs are co-analgesics:
1 Clonidine
2 Doxapram
3 Baclofen
4 Carbimazole
5 Carbamazepine

Page 773
The following are bad prognostic indicators in back pain:
1 Negative family history
2 Long history
3 Polypharmacy
4 Modest diet
5 Physical fitness

The following are related to chronic low back pain:
1 Neck problems
2 Introversion
3 Obesity
4 High stress levels
5 Smoking

Page 775
The 'learned pain syndrome' is characterised by:
1 Dramatisation of complaints
2 Drunkenness
3 Drug misuse with frequently changed prescriptions
4 Dependency helplessness and parasitism
5 Disability in social life

Page 776
Various types of migraine may be precipitated by:
1 Red wine
2 Stress
3 Cold hands

The following factors modify non-acute pain:
1 False (alkalosis is a result of pain, not a cause)
2 True (antidepressives often used in non-acute pain)
3 True (loss of hope is a feature of 'total pain')
4 False   *it does ! men suffer more*
5 True (e.g. migraine in the morning)

The following drugs are co-analgesics:
1 True (potentiates analgesics and local anaesthetics)
2 False (used for reversing respiratory depression)
3 True (an antispasmodic)
4 False (an antithyroid drug)
5 True (also anti-epileptic)

The following are bad prognostic indicators in back pain:
1 False
2 True
3 True
4 False
5 False (unless pursued to a violent degree)

The following are related to chronic low back pain:
1 True
2 True
3 True
4 True
5 True

The 'learned pain syndrome' is characterised by:
1 True
2 False (not related)
3 True
4 True
5 True

Various types of migraine may be precipitated by:
1 True
2 True (stress management is part of the treatment)
3 True (easily managed with gloves)

4 Bright lights
5 Starvation

Page 776
The pain of nerve entrapment:
1 May be a burning pain
2 May be a shooting pain
3 Associated with anorexia
4 Associated with local weakness and wasting
5 Causes loss of local sensation

Page 777
Postherpetic neuralgia:
1 Occurs in between 10 and 20% of cases of herpes zoster
2 Is uncommon under the age of 40
3 May be prevented by i.v. guanethidine block
4 Is related to the severity of the rash
5 Is relieved by light touch

4 True (photophobia is also a result of a migraine attack)
5 True (preanaesthetic starvation may require glucose
administration: migraine may also cause a craving for
sweet foods)

The pain of nerve entrapment:
1 True
2 True
3 False
4 True
5 True

Postherpetic neuralgia:
1 True
2 True (mainly a disease of the older patient)
3 True (if done early in the herpes attack)
4 False
5 False (triggered by light touch)

Section 6:
Cardiorespiratory intensive care

Chapters 22 (Paediatric), 28 and 30

In the special care baby unit (SCBU):
1 Pneumothorax is common
2 Bacteriology swabs are taken more than once daily
3 Ambient temperature is 20°C
4 Feeding is carried out 6 hourly
5 Infection is indicated by pyrexia

In the neonate:
1 Apgar score of 6 is an indication for intubation and IPPV
2 Rapid infusion of Haemaccel may precipitate intracranial haemorrhage
3 Babies with low Apgar scores are likely to be volume depleted
4 Nose to mid-trachea distance in a term infant is 10 cm
5 IPPV rate of 30–35 per minute is usual

The neonatal cardiovascular system:
1 Ductal patency can be maintained with PGE_1 or PGE_2 infused at $0.1\,\mu g/kg/min$
2 The ductus can be constricted by indomethacin
3 Indomethacin may cause platelet dysfunction
4 Indomethacin may worsen renal failure
5 Right to left shunt indicates worsening pulmonary disease

Monitoring and therapy in the neonate:
1 PaO_2 is kept above $100\,mmHg$ ($13.3\,kPa$)
2 Vascular access is essentially similar to the adult
3 PaO_2 may be measured by transcutaneous electrodes
4 Hyperventilation is used to reduce neonatal pulmonary hypertension
5 Blood glucose is measured daily

Page 789 and Chapter 22 (Paediatric and Neurosurgical)
Paediatric intensive care:
1 Core–toe temperature gradient is an index of cardiac output
2 Core–toe temperature gradient is an index of peripheral vascular tone
3 Pulmonary circulation is less reactive than the adult

4 Positive Kernig's sign is characteristic of infant bacterial meningitis
5 Cerebral perfusion pressure is maintained above $50\,mmHg$ in the head-injured child

In the special care baby unit (SCBU):
1 True (may be detected by transillumination of the chest)
2 True (greater infection risk due to immature immune system)
3 False (36.5°C in incubator or under radiator)
4 False (2 hourly or continuous)
5 False (febrile response is often lacking)

In the neonate:
1 False (Apgar scores of 1–2)

2 True
3 True
4 True
5 True

The neonatal cardiovascular system:

1 True
2 True
3 True
4 True (a reversible effect)
5 True (applies to the majority of SCBU patients)

Monitoring and therapy in the neonate:
1 False (50–80 mmHg (6.6–10.6 kPa) to prevent retinopathy)
2 True (umbilical artery and vein are also used in the newborn)
3 True (as is $PaCO_2$)

4 True (to $PaCO_2$ 25–30 mmHg, 3.3–4.0 kPa)
5 False (much more frequently)

Paediatric intensive care:
1 True (inverse relationship)

2 True (direct relationship)
3 False (much more reactive and severe pulmonary
         vasoconstriction is not uncommon)

4 False (and fever, stiff neck etc. are also often absent)

5 True (and ICP monitoring should be readily available)

In the critically ill child:
1 Inappropriate ADH secretion does not occur
2 Subglottic stenosis occurs in Down's syndrome
3 IPPV rate of 35 per minute is usual for children
4 Severe trauma causes acute gastric dilation
5 Thermoregulation is not a problem

Page 790
The high dependency units are appropriate for:
1 IPPV
2 Management of extradural catheters
3 Treatment of septic shock syndrome
4 Management of severe pain
5 Management of massive haemorrhage

Page 794
Shock may be caused by:
1 Hypothyroidism
2 Acute Addison's disease
3 Gram negative septicaemia
4 Sudden deceleration
5 Surgical traction on gall bladder

Hypovolaemia may be caused by:
1 Dehydration
2 Fractured pelvis
3 Burns
4 Diarrhoea
5 Frusemide 20 mg

Page 795
In cardiogenic shock due to myocardial infarction:
1 The severity is related to cardiac rhythm
2 Prognosis is better if septal defect occurs
3 Papillary rupture makes it worse
4 Opioids are contraindicated
5 Mesenteric perfusion is improved by dopamine

Pages 798–800
Drugs used in shock:
1 Dobutamine acts as a relatively pure inotrope
2 Dopexamine tends to reduce renal blood flow
3 Phosphodiesterase inhibitors have a long half-life
4 Nitroprusside releases cyanide only when administered in excess

In the critically ill child:
1 False (it is common)
2 True (it is common)
3 False (15–20 is usual)
4 True (very common)
5 False (a constant problem)

The high dependency units are appropriate for:
1 True (but only very short-term – a few hours)
2 True
3 False (this is intensive therapy)
4 True
5 False (this is intensive therapy)

Shock may be caused by:
1 False
2 True (hypotension and failed tissue perfusion)
3 True (see Chapter 33)
4 True (in motor and aerospace accidents)
5 True (due to a vagal reflex with bradycardia)

Hypovolaemia may be caused by:
1 True (from whatever cause)
2 True
3 True (due to plasma loss)
4 True (due to water and electrolyte losses)
5 False

In cardiogenic shock due to myocardial infarction:
1 True (arrhythmias worsen 'pump failure')
2 False (much worse due to intra-cardiac shunting)
3 True (valvular incompetence occurs)
4 False (still needed for pain)
5 True (renal perfusion is also improved)

Drugs used in shock:
1 True (cardiac beta-1 stimulant)
2 False (splanchnic and renal vasodilator)
3 True (e.g. repeat doses every 3–6 hours for enoximone)
4 False (each molecule releases 5 cyanide radicals)

5 The metabolism of cyanide is enhanced by sodium thiosulphate

Page 800
Vasodilation is caused by:
1 Trinitrotoluidine
2 Glyceryl trinitrate
3 Nifedipine
4 Methylamphetamine
5 Phentolamine

In a patient with acute myocardial infarction you should:
1 Give diclofenac i.v.
2 Give GTN i.v.
3 Avoid giving opioids
4 Give atropine unless the pulse rate is over 100 per minute

5 Avoid more than 28% oxygen

Page 801
The following are used in the treatment of acute myocardial infarction:
1 Ciprofloxacin
2 Streptomycin
3 Aspirin
4 Atenolol
5 Ketamine

5 True (it is used as an antidote, dose 5–10 g i.v.)

Vasodilation is caused by:
1 False (this is an explosive)
2 True (sublingual dose 0.3–1 mg)
3 True (a peripheral calcium antagonist, dose 10 mg)
4 False (a vasoconstrictor)
5 True (an alpha 1 & 2 blocker, dose 1–10 mg i.v.)

In a patient with acute myocardial infarction you should:
1 False (not currently available)
2 False (sublingually is a safer and effective route)
3 False (they are often needed)
4 False (only for the sinus bradycardia seen especially after inferior infarction)
5 False (oxygen is very important)

The following are used in the treatment of acute myocardial infarction:
1 False (an antibiotic)
2 False (streptokinase is used early)
3 True (very effective)
4 True (if not contra-indicated, may limit infarct size)
5 False (a good analgesic but a vasoconstrictor)

30 Respiratory failure

Page 803
The following can indicate respiratory failure in the adult:
1 Ten words per breath
2 Cyanosis
3 Tachypnoea greater than 30 per minute
4 Borborygmi
5 Grimacing and alar flaring

The following indicate respiratory inadequacy:
1 $PaCO_2$ of 4.5 kPa
2 PaO_2 of 8 kPa
3 FEV_1 of 1 litre
4 Standard bicarbonate of 35 mmol/l
5 Pre-tibial oedema

Page 806
The following may complicate IPPV in the intensive care unit:
1 Atelectasis
2 Peripheral oedema
3 Colitis
4 Hallucinations
5 Chest infection

Page 808
Tracheostomy may be complicated by:
1 Tracheal dilation
2 Tracheal stenosis
3 Carotid haemorrhage
4 Increased deadspace
5 Pneumothorax

Page 811
An asthmatic patient would be likely to need IPPV if:
1 PaO_2 was more than 9 kPa
2 Polyuria is occurring
3 There was bradycardia
4 Pulsus paradoxus is greater than 40 mmHg
5 Pneumothorax has precipitated the crisis

Adult respiratory distress syndrome (ARDS):
1 Is primarily a disease of the airways
2 Is primarily a disorder of the blood vessels
3 Hypercapnia is an early finding

The following can indicate respiratory failure in the adult:
1 False (less than 2 words per breath)
2 True (PaO_2 less than about 8 kPa)
3 True
4 False
5 True (indicating dyspnoea)

The following indicate respiratory inadequacy:
1 False (this indicates mild hyperventilation)
2 True (cyanosis level)
3 True (this is a critically low level in an adult)
4 True (metabolic response to respiratory acidosis)
5 False (a sign of myxoedema)

The following may complicate IPPV in the intensive care unit:
1 True
2 True (worsened by PEEP)
3 False (although this may be caused by concurrent drugs)
4 True
5 True

Tracheostomy may be complicated by:
1 True (due to cuff pressure)
2 True (later, due to mucosal scarring)
3 True (due to ulceration locally)
4 False (decreased deadspace)
5 True (rarely)

An asthmatic patient would be likely to need IPPV if:
1 False (less than 9 kPa)
2 False (oliguria is a relative indication)
3 False (increasing tachycardia is a relative indication for IPPV)
4 True
5 True (X-ray and chest drainage will be required)

Adult respiratory distress syndrome (ARDS):
1 False
2 True (endothelial damage in pulmonary capillaries)
3 False (hypoxia is the classic presenting sign)

135

4 May be caused by acute pancreatitis
5 Is an indication for hydrocortisone

ARDS:
1 Its pathogenesis involves tumour necrosis factor
2 Raises right ventricular output
3 Is cured by extra-corporeal membrane oxygenation
4 Is associated with a high plasma colloid osmotic pressure
5 Causes increased lung lymphatic flow

Pages 812–813
The following are predictors of survival in ARDS:
1 Serum lactate less than 25 mmol/l
2 A high serum elastase
3 The patient is in the older age group
4 A greater number of organs involved
5 Low myeloperoxidase levels

Page 814
In tetanus:
1 Paralysis occurs
2 Laryngeal obstruction occurs
3 Autonomic failure occurs
4 Beta blockade is needed
5 Tracheal suction lowers the CVP

Page 815
Acute inflammatory epiglottitis:
1 Is caused by *Haemophilus influenzae* type B
2 May be visible on X-ray
3 Is often accompanied by drooling in children
4 Is helped by breathing 21% oxygen in helium
5 Is an indication for antibiotics

Page 816
Acute laryngotracheitis in children:
1 Has an insidious onset
2 The child drools
3 Lung collapse is a frequent complication
4 Pulmonary oedema may occur
5 Tracheostomy is indicated

4 True (the cause is often remote from the lung)
5 False (of no value and may make things worse)

ARDS:
1 True (anti-TNF antibody has been tried as therapy)
2 False (causes right ventricular failure)
3 False (this may buy time but is not curative)
4 False (a low plasma colloid osmotic pressure)
5 True (increased lung water; the lungs weigh > 1000 g)

The following are predictors of survival in ARDS:
1 False (serum lactate less than 2.5 mmol/l)
2 False (a low serum elastase)
3 False (younger age group)
4 False (this worsens prognosis)
5 True (less than 10 ng/ml is normal)

In tetanus:
1 False (prolonged spastic convulsions)
2 True (due to muscle spasm)
3 False (autonomic overactivity is a problem)
4 True (to control sympathetic effects on the heart)
5 False (raises the CVP dramatically)

Acute inflammatory epiglottitis:
1 True
2 True (but waiting for X-ray may cause critical delay)
3 True (drooling and sitting up are classic signs)
4 True (has low density)
5 True (ampicillin, chloramphenicol or cephalosporins)

Acute laryngotracheitis in children:
1 False (frequently in a matter of hours)
2 False (this is a sign of acute epiglottitis)
3 True
4 True
5 False (to be avoided if possible)

Page 818

Oxygen flux:

1 Is a function of cardiac output
2 Is a function of haemoglobin level
3 Meets the oxygen demand of the body
4 Is a determinant of outcome in septic shock syndrome
5 Is $SaO_2 (\%/100) \times 1.34 \times$ Hb (g/ml) $\times$ cardiac output (ml/min)

Page 819

Hypoxia:

1 Directly stimulates the respiratory centre
2 Causes pulmonary vasodilation
3 Stimulates diuresis
4 Is a coronary vasoconstrictor
5 Shortens the PR interval in the ECG

Changing to breathing pure oxygen:

1 Interferes with CO_2 transport

2 Constricts cerebral arteries
3 Constricts pulmonary arteries
4 Causes patchy opacities on chest X-ray
5 Helps dissociate carbon monoxide from HbCO

Page 822

High air-flow oxygen-enrichment (HAFOE) masks:

1 Utilise the venturi principle
2 Have small openings in the sides
3 Have total inflow into the mask of about 30 l/min
4 Have outflow up to 60 l/min
5 Entrainment ratio is independent of oxygen flow

Page 823

Oxygen concentrators:

1 Use an aluminosilicate
2 Absorb oxygen on to zeolite
3 Produce a continuous flow of gas
4 Are independent of electricity
5 Produce pure oxygen

Oxygen flux:
1 True
2 True
3 False (an O_2 debt may build up)
4 True (an attempt is made to deliver more O_2 to tissues)
5 True

Hypoxia:
1 False (indirectly via the carotid and aortic bodies)
2 False (causes pulmonary vasoconstriction)
3 False (causes renal failure)
4 False (coronary vasodilator)
5 False (lengthens PR interval)

Changing to breathing pure oxygen:
1 True (CO_2 is carried as carbamino compounds on reduced Hb; but this interference is only significant under hyperbaric conditions)
2 True
3 False (dilates them)
4 True (after some days)
5 True (reduces half-life of HbCO to 50–60 min)

High air-flow oxygen-enrichment (HAFOE) masks:
1 True
2 False (large openings for exhaling)
3 True (equals maximum inspiratory flow rate)
4 True (inflow plus expiratory flow)
5 True (but total inflow should be set to 30 l/min)

Oxygen concentrators:
1 True (zeolite)
2 False (absorb nitrogen)
3 False (zeolite must be purged intermittently)
4 False (they need electricity)
5 False (produce 94% oxygen, and concentrate atmospheric argon)

Page 823
In hyperbaric oxygen therapy:
1 At 2 atmospheres 100 ml plasma contains 4.2 ml O_2
2 'Bends' may occur on rapid compression
3 Decompression causes mist formation
4 Venous blood is nearly fully oxygenated
5 Is an effective treatment for ischaemia in acute vasculitis

In hyperbaric oxygen therapy:
1 True
2 False (on decompression)
3 True (due to fall of temperature)
4 True (dissolved O_2 alone virtually meets tissue needs)
5 True (tissue oxygenation can be restored)

31 Resuscitation

In basic cardiac life-support:
1 5 cardiac compressions to 1 ventilation is the correct ratio
2 The femoral pulse is found at the anterior superior iliac spine
3 The precordial thump is given after the patient arrives in casualty
4 External chest compressions are performed on a line between the nipples
5 External chest compressions are performed over the middle third of the sternum

Tracheal intubation in advanced cardiac life-support (ACLS):
1 May make the head-injured patient vomit
2 Requires the fibreoptic laryngoscope
3 Requires the straight-bladed laryngoscope in infants
4 Intubation and IPPV may worsen a pneumothorax
5 Is avoided in stridor

The following arrhythmias may mimic ventricular tachycardia:
1 Supraventricular tachycardia (SVT) with aberrant conduction
2 Wolff–Parkinson–White syndrome
3 Wenckebach phenomenon
4 'Torsade de pointes'
5 Ventricular fibrillation

If the ECG shows sudden asystole, would you:
1 Give a 300 J DC shock?
2 Give 50 mmol of sodium bicarbonate?
3 Give adrenaline 1 mg i.v.?
4 Give a precordial thump?
5 Check the ECG electrodes?

Electro-mechanical dissociation is seen in:
1 Cardiac arrest due to haemorrhage
2 Cardiac tamponade
3 Patients with ECG activity but no pulses
4 Massive pulmonary embolus
5 Acute myocardial infarction

Drug administration during ACLS:
1 A leg vein cannula is the route of choice

2 An arm vein cannula is the route of choice

3 The endotracheal route is the route of choice

In basic cardiac life-support:
1 True (unless you are single handed)
2 False (mid-inguinal point; lateral edge of the pubic hair)
3 False (immediately after the arrest)

4 False (the nipples are very variable in position)

5 True (sternal length is checked before starting)

Tracheal intubation in advanced cardiac life-support (ACLS):
1 True (a brief general anaesthetic with relaxant is needed)
2 False (takes too long)
3 True (preferable, but not essential)
4 True (air forced out of lung into pleura)
5 False (a smaller tube is usually needed, e.g. less than 6 mm)

The following arrhythmias may mimic ventricular tachycardia:
1 True
2 False (although it may cause SVT)
3 False (not a tachyarrhythmia)
4 True (a type of VT)
5 True (but the treatment is the same)

If the ECG shows sudden asystole, would you:
1 False (conversion to VF needed first)
2 False (only if there is metabolic acidosis)
3 True (to convert to VF)
4 True (an initial treatment)
5 True (a disconnected electrode gives a straight-line trace)

Electro-mechanical dissociation is seen in:
1 True (massive infusion urgently needed)
2 True (treated by pericardial aspiration)
3 True (this defines it)
4 True (physical blockage of circulation)
5 True (and carries a very bad prognosis)

Drug administration during ACLS:
1 False (takes too long to circulate unless there is absolutely no
      other route)
2 False (drugs may take 2–4 min to circulate, but may suffice until
      a central line is set up)
3 False (an alternative route for adrenaline and atropine, but not
      for other drugs, e.g. $CaCl_2$)

4 An intracardiac cannula is the route of choice
5 A central venous cannula is the route of choice

Page 832
In near-drowning:
1 It is important to know if the water was fresh or salt

2 If the patient has been under water for 10 min, treatment is not started
3 'Secondary drowning' does not occur after 1 hour
4 Antibiotics are needed
5 The pupils are a good prognostic indicator

In near-drowning:
1 The lungs can be emptied of water by a steep head-down position
2 Pulmonary oedema may be a complication
3 Hyperthermia is a feature
4 Steroids are often administered
5 Intravenous glucose is given

4 False (causes physical damage to the heart)
5 True

In near-drowning:
1 True (different pathophysiology, although many aspects of
       treatment are similar)

2 False (limit is 30 min)
3 False (may occur more than a day later)
4 True
5 False (they may be dilated with cold)

In near-drowning:

1 False (IPPV is indicated)
2 True (haemodilution and cardiac failure)
3 False (hypothermia; most drownings occur in cold water)
4 True
5 True (hypoglycaemia is common)

32 Trauma and multiple injuries

Pages 835–840
In accidents, the following have serious significance:
1 Fall of more than 20 feet
2 Being hit by motor vehicle
3 Ejection from a moving vehicle
4 Being in a car impact at < 10 mph
5 Death of a person in the same vehicle

Poor prognosis in trauma is indicated by:
1 Facial burns
2 Penetrating injury of thorax
3 Shock index of 0.5
4 Trauma score of 8
5 APACHE score of 5

In head injuries, the following are indicators for intensive care:
1 Respiratory rate of less than 10/min

2 Unconsciousness
3 Bradycardia
4 CPK in the CSF of more than 150 units/l
5 Associated double limb fractures

Page 849
APACHE scoring:
1 0 is at the extreme of abnormality
2 Involves serum chloride levels
3 Makes use of TISS
4 Scores greater in old age
5 Immuno-suppression raises the 'chronic health evaluation' score

Page 851
Poisoning:
1 Diarrhoea should be encouraged in mushroom poisoning
2 Fluids should be restricted in mushroom poisoning
3 Chlorpromazine is an antidote in early paraquat poisoning
4 Charcoal haemoperfusion helps in organophosphorus poisoning
5 The dose of activated charcoal is 1 g/kg

In accidents, the following have serious significance:
1 True
2 True
3 True
4 False (> 20 mph)
5 True

Poor prognosis in trauma is indicated by:
1 True
2 True
3 False (pulse rate/systolic pressure of 0.5 is normal)
4 True
5 False (over 20 is very serious)

In head injuries, the following are indicators for intensive care:
1 True (to prevent hypoxic brain damage secondary to
        hypoventilation)
2 True
3 True (may indicate cerebral compression)
4 True (indicates cerebral damage)
5 True (major blood loss)

APACHE scoring:
1 False (0 is normal)
2 False (involves Na; K; pH and creatinine)
3 False (uses Glasgow coma score)
4 True
5 True

Poisoning:
1 True (to remove the toxins)
2 False (aggressive fluid replacement)
3 True (it reduces pulmonary uptake)
4 True
5 True (given by nasogastric tube)

Page 352
In carbon monoxide (CO) poisoning:
1 The primary therapy is oxygen
2 Oxygen has no effect on the half-life of HbCO
3 30% HbCO is an indication for hyperbaric oxygenation
4 The absorption spectrum of HbCO is about 600 nm
5 High lactate levels indicate a good prognosis

In carbon monoxide (CO) poisoning:
1 True
2 False (it reduces it to less than 60 min)
3 True
4 True
5 False (low lactate levels)

33 Sepsis and the septic syndrome

Page 855
Features of septic shock include:
1 Bradycardia
2 Polyuria
3 Fever
4 Hypothermia
5 Early hypercarbia

The following are seen in septic shock syndrome:
1 Infection
2 Negative blood cultures
3 Coagulopathy
4 Coma
5 Anaemia

Monitoring in septic shock syndrome:
1 Hypotension is common
2 Reduced metabolic rate is seen
3 Myeloperoxidase levels are less than 10 ng/ml
4 SVR is greater than 1,000 dynes.sec.cm^{-5}
5 Pulmonary vascular resistance (PVR) is low

Page 856
Survival in septic shock is better when:
1 Raised oxygen delivery increases oxygen consumption
2 Renal function is maintained
3 The patient is over 65 years
4 Integrity of gut wall is maintained
5 Frank–Starling curve shifts to the right

Features of septic shock include:
1 False (tachycardia)
2 False (oliguria and renal failure)
3 True (greater than 38.5°C)
4 True (less than 35.5°C)
5 False (hypoxia is the characteristic sign)

The following are seen in septic shock syndrome:
1 True (but can be non-infective in origin!)
2 False (frequently positive)
3 True (a common complication)
4 True (indicating cerebral involvement)
5 True (indicating haemorrhage or bone marrow involvement)

Monitoring in septic shock syndrome:
1 True
2 False (raised to more than 40 kcal/sq.m/hr)
3 False (more than 200 ng/ml)
4 False (less than 800 dynes.sec.cm^{-5})
5 False (PVR greater than 200 dynes.sec.cm^{-5})

Survival in septic shock is better when:
1 True
2 True (1 and 2 are important aims of treatment)
3 False (young patients survive better)
4 True (preventing endotoxin absorption)
5 False (shifts left and up)

34 Nutrition

Pages 867–871
Normal daily nutritional requirements for a 70 kg man include:
1 Protein 200 g
2 Between 2,000 and 2,500 kcal
3 Sodium 100 mmol
4 Pantothenic acid
5 Zinc

Parenteral nutrition:
1 Must be given through a central venous catheter

2 Protein is given as a solution of D-amino acids
3 Fat provides the most calories per g of substrate
4 Muscle breakdown can exceed 0.5 kg/day in a catabolic patient
5 Protein must be accompanied by another source of calories to allow its best usage

Page 867
Nutritional support is indicated in:
1 Polyphagy
2 Major sepsis
3 Preoperative malnutrition
4 Increased skinfold thickness
5 Coma

Page 868
Complications of enteral nutritional support include:
1 Cholecystitis
2 Diarrhoea
3 Pulmonary aspiration
4 Bone marrow suppression
5 Oliguria

Pages 869–870
Intravenous nutrients:
1 1 litre of isotonic glucose contains 8.4 MJ of energy
2 The liver cannot handle a large amino acid load and so it is not possible to replace all of the 15 g/day of nitrogen lost in a moderately catabolic patient
3 More CO_2 is produced per calorie of energy if glucose is the only substrate
4 Fat emulsions are made isotonic by adding glycerol
5 Vitamins in the B group degrade on exposure to light

Normal daily nutritional requirements for a 70 kg man include:
1 False (70 g)
2 True (8.4 to 10.5 MJ)
3 True
4 True
5 True (zinc depletion may cause acrodermatitis enteropathica)

Parenteral nutrition:
1 False (fat emulsions and some amino acid solutions can be given peripherally)
2 False (L-isomers are used)
3 True (9 kcal/g, carbohydrate and protein are 4 kcal/g)
4 True

5 True (otherwise protein is used for calorie consumption)

Nutritional support is indicated in:
1 False (indicated in anorexia)
2 True (these patients need enhanced calorie intake)
3 True (and helps postoperative recovery)
4 False (decreased skinfold thickness)
5 True (unable to eat normally)

Complications of enteral nutritional support include:
1 True (due to alteration of gut flora)
2 True (treated by codeine)
3 True
4 False
5 False

Intravenous nutrients:
1 False (only 840 kJ or 200 kcal)

2 False (up to about 24 g N/day can be given)

3 True (glucose gives the highest respiratory quotient)
4 True
5 True

Page 872

Parenteral nutrition may cause:

1 Cholecystitis
2 Pneumothorax
3 Hyperosmolar syndrome
4 Hypoglycaemia
5 A shift to the left of the O_2 dissociation curve

Parenteral nutrition may cause:
1 True (due to alteration of gut flora)
2 True (from central line insertion)
3 True (due to hypertonic glucose)
4 False (hyperglycaemia if insulin is not given)
5 True (due to phosphate deficiency)